THE NEW
NATUROPATHIC DIET

THE NEW
NATUROPATHIC DIET

How to Manage Your Weight, Prevent Illness and Achieve Optimum Health

PENNY KENDALL-REED, ND
with STEPHEN REED, MD

WINDING
STAIR
PRESS

The publisher acknowledges the support of the Book
Publishing Industry Development Program,
Department of Canadian Heritage,
Government of Canada.

The publisher does not advocate the use of any particular treatment program, but believes that the information presented in this book should be available to the public. The nutritional, medical, and health information presented in this book is based on the research, training, and personal experiences of the author, and is true and complete to the best of the author's knowledge. However, this book is intended only as an informative guide for those wishing to know more about good health. It is not intended to replace or countermand the advice given by the reader's physician. Because there is always some risk involved, the author and publisher are not responsible for any adverse effects or consequences resulting from any of the suggestions made in this book. And because each person and each situation is unique, the author and the publisher urge the reader to consult with a qualified health care professional before using any procedure where there is a question as to its appropriateness. It is a sign of wisdom, not cowardice, to seek a second or third opinion.

ISBN 1-55082-302-7

Design by Sari Naworynski.
Front cover photograph by Hillendale Studios.
Back Cover photograph by José Crespo.

Printed and bound in Canada by Webcom.

Published by Winding Stair Press
An imprint of Stewart House Publishing Inc.
195 Allstate Parkway
Markham, Ontario
L3R 4T8
and
1180 Medical Court, Suite A
Carmel, Indiana
46032

CONTENTS

PRINCIPLES OF THE NATUROPATHIC DIET

We must train our body to use food as fuel rather than storing it as fat, enabling permanent weight loss, increasing our energy level, and preventing chronic diet-related diseases.

Weight Loss

Increase dietary protein to 15-25 grams per meal

Eat unlimited salad vegetables (low glycemic carbohydrates)

Limit or restrict high glycemic (high sugar content) vegetables, legumes, and fruits

Eliminate simple carbohydrates (bread, rice, potatoes, refined sugar) and alcohol

Enjoy limited condiments

Weight Maintenance

Maintain dietary protein level of 15-25 grams per meal

Reintroduce, slowly, some limited, resticted, and forbidden carbohydrates

Aim for a 1:1 ratio of protein to carbohydrates

Adjust ratio for hyperinsulemia symptoms

Nutritional Supplementation

Supplement diet with required minerals and vitamins

Enhance weight loss with herbs, minerals, fatty acids, lipids

Detoxification

Eat certified organic foods
Detoxify body with herbs and clean food

Augmentation

Augment diet with protein rich soy foods for beneficial
phytoestrogen effects

INTRODUCTION

The Desire to Diet and the Drive to Eat More

E ach morning, many of us wake thinking that today just might be the day to begin a diet to lose weight. Our intentions are good, motivation is high, but as we begin to prepare our first meal, we are bombarded with a multitude of food choices that psychologically and physiologically impair our desire and ability to lose weight. The majority of food options available to us not only force our bodies to store our meal as fat, but rapidly result in low blood sugar levels, making us feel hungry once again. We feel the need to eat more food, defeating our 'good' diet intentions.

This drive to eat more is the primary cause of the weight problem North Americans and Europeans are facing, which in turn is responsible in part for many related health problems. The number of overweight people in America has risen each year since the late 1960s; according to the research of the American Dietetic Association, in the overall population there has been an average increase of 13% body fat. Never before has society been so dangerously overweight.

With the addition of these extra pounds, the risk of diabetes, heart disease, high cholesterol, and hypertension increases greatly.

The problem lies in what we eat and how we eat it – in our 'diet' or nutrition practices. The function of our body can be compared to that of a car. If we put clean gas into our cars, the car will travel faster and longer, be more efficient, and spend less time in the repair shop. If we put 'good food' into our bodies, we, too, will function optimally, with greater vitality and with fewer visits to the doctor. But if we fill our body with nutrient poor food or poorly balanced food, the result may well be disease.

Being overweight is historically a rather recent phenomenon. If we look back through time, humans have been quite lean. In the beginning, we ate simply what was available, a diet consisting of meat or game, berries or fruit and plants. Evolution-wise, this is what the human body is designed for, and these are the food types that the body prefers. When we developed convenience crops and processed foods, we laid the foundations for an industry that has never stopped growing. Wheat, rice, and other farmed foods were cultivated and processed. They could easily be grown and stored with little work, providing a reliable source of calories. Wheat and rice soon expanded into pasta and ready-made meals all containing many nutritionally empty calories and a disproportionate amount of carbohydrate. Most convenience foods that are easily available today contain an incorrect or unhealthy ratio of nutrients that send a message to our bodies to store fat. This imbalanced fuel has slowly forced our bodies to store more fat and hold onto the fat that we already have, creating the overweight society we see today.

Diet Trends

Many different 'diets' have been developed over time to try to slow down or stop our ever-growing weight problem. Diet trends come and go, but, despite varying degrees of initial success, the calorie-deprivation, low-fat, and high-carbohydrate programs have not been shown to be consistently effective over time. Even the latest high-protein diets have some serious shortcomings.

Calorie-reduced diets flaunt their rapid weight loss, in some cases up to five pounds each week. This type of weight loss, however, causes other problems, which make maintenance of the reduced weight very difficult. Excessively rapid weight loss stimulates production of an enzyme known as lipoprotein lipase, which forces our bodies to store more fat. Ultimately, this slows down our metabolic rate and therefore slows down weight loss. These diets at this stage mimic starvation and force the body to hold onto whatever food it is given. As well, the food groups chosen in these diets are imbalanced and disproportionately high in carbohydrates.

With the advent of the low-fat diet came the theory that if you want to lose fat, don't eat it! Dean Ornish's diet is one such low fat diet. Not only is this diet difficult to follow due to its nutritional restrictions, but the extreme reduction in fat leaves individuals permanently hungry. It may also have a detrimental effect on the body. While low fat diets are very successful in lowering LDL ("bad cholesterol") levels, they also reduce HDL ("good cholesterol") levels quite dramatically. Certain studies show that these low fat diets may even *increase* the risk of heart disease by lowering HDL levels too far. If you eliminate all the foods with fat in them, all that is left are grains, fruits, and vegetables, essentially another version of a high-carbohydrate diet that, as we shall see, will eventually fail.

Removing 'good' unsaturated fats from our diet is also dangerous for our health, for these fats are integral to the construction of cell membranes and the regulation of hormones, among other essential bodily functions.

Eating just a diet high in carbohydrates seems to be a logical solution to our weight-loss problem. These ingested carbohydrates are low in fat, low in cholesterol, and therefore lower in calories. So it seems to make sense to eat carbohydrates primarily, such as pasta, rice, or potatoes, a regime promoted by *Fit For Life* and the Canada Food Guide, for example. Unfortunately, once the carbohydrates are ingested, this picture almost reverses due to the different hormonal secretion that occurs in response to a high carbohydrate meal. There is, in fact, an increase in fat production and storage as well as a rise in blood triglyceride and cholesterol levels. These plain and simple carbohydrates become havoc-wreaking substrates that damage the body. Sadly, this diet was advocated before any sound clinical data was collected. On paper, these foods looked good, but in reality they have only increased our weight problem, accentuating the process of fat storage that we are now trying to reverse. A high carbohydrate diet has also increased our risk of diet-related diseases.

In a study of the French population, who have far less obesity and cardiovascular disease than North Americans, Dr Michel Montignac was one of the first to postulate that carbohydrate, rather than fat, is the crucial component in weight gain. He also questioned the effect of low calorie diets. Montignac's suggestion that the secretion of insulin could be tightly controlled simply by consuming only those carbohydrates with a low glycemic (sugar) index inspired Dr Morrison Bethea, Head of Cardiac Surgery at Mercy-Baptist Hospital in New-Orleans, to conduct studies on the insulin-cholesterol connection. By following a diet consisting of low glycemic carbohydrates, total cholesterol levels were reduced by 20% to 30% in most individuals. Dr. Jennifer Marks at the University of Miami performed another series of studies on insulin resistance. She recognized that insulin resistance was characterized by glucose intolerance, an increase in cholesterol and triglycerides, high blood pressure, and obesity. It is well known that any one of these conditions alone greatly increases the risk of heart disease. However, further studies showed that the risk increased dramatically in the presence of more than one condition. This was demonstrated by a PROCAM (Prospective Cardiovascular Munster) study of 2,754 men between the ages of 40 and 60: if a person had diabetes *or* high blood pressure alone, then the risk of a heart attack was 2.5 times greater than that of a normal individual, but when an individual had both diabetes and high blood pressure, the risk increased 8 times. Dr. David Brown has shown that excessive insulin levels stimulate growth of the cells lining arteries, which, in turn, decreases the available space for the blood to flow. This ultimately increases blood pressure. High insulin levels also instruct the kidneys to hold onto salt, again increasing blood pressure.

If high-carbohydrate diets are so ineffective and potentially dangerous, what about the new protein diets? The focus of many of the high-protein diets is simply to lose weight, quickly. They are not concerned with what type of weight is lost as long as a reduction is seen on the scales. Unfortunately, much of the loss is from muscle rather than fat, but maintaining muscle in the body is essential for permanent weight loss. Muscle cells contain components called mitochondria, which can be considered the 'calorie furnaces' or 'power houses' for the body. These cells burn up fat and create more energy. The more muscle you have, the more fat burning potential exists. Despite the potential for being effective in reducing weight in the short term, these protein diets are often so complex that the average person finds them too difficult to follow for any length of time. In addition, some are so restrictive of other food groups or imbalanced that they impose a separate set of problems, such as ketosis, which can damage the kidneys.

Several high protein diets have become popular. Programs such as the Carbohydrate Addict's Diet advocated by Rachael and Richard Heller, Dr Atkins' New Diet, and the Protein Power Plan diet developed by Michael and Mary Eades are biochemically well-grounded. Their premise of reducing insulin secretion so that we do not store our food as fat is sound. While they provide a foundation on which to build an effective protein-based diet, they lack many nutrients and are quite deficient in valuable carbohydrates such as fruits and vegetables. These nutrients are vital to the growth and well-being of the body. In addition, if the carbohydrate content of the diet is too low in relation to protein, the body will assume a starvation state called ketosis. This process is essentially the body's emergency response to lack of food. Its purpose is survival at the expense of health. Ketosis results in symptoms such as nausea, dehydration, light-headedness, and bad breath. Toxic effects to the body include kidney damage. Ketosis may be fatal to diabetics and to the fetus in pregnancy.

With respect to weight reduction, ketosis results in weight loss due to dehydration and loss of muscle tissue. Not only is this harmful to the body but ultimately causes increased weight gain. Protein ingestion in ketosis can stimulate insulin release to convert the amino acids into fat. Also studies have shown that ketogenic diets alter fat cells to make them more hungry for fat storage.

Compliance with many of the protein diets is low due to their dietary restrictions. The Atkins' Diet outlaws condiments and dressings, leaving the allowable food quite bland. Both the Atkins' Diet and the Protein Power Plan involve complex measurements and calculations which are difficult to follow. The average busy individual has only 30 minutes to prepare and eat a meal. The Carbohydrate Addict's Diet offers a reward meal every day, which not only slows the weight loss process but makes dieters feel as if they are being deprived all day long so that a "reward" is then needed. A program of deprivation followed by reward is not a healthy approach to weight loss maintenance, nor likely to result in a lifelong dietary change. Barry Sears' The Zone is a good *maintenance* diet, but it can take many months to see any significant weight loss.

While the concept of a protein-based diet is central to safe and successful weight-loss and cardiovascular health, there are many other factors which need to be incorporated. These include the addition of soy to the diet, the importance of organic foodstuffs, the need to detoxify the body, and the inclusion of naturopathic supplements to enhance the rate of weight loss, safely. There are no diets currently available that include these principles.

The Naturopathic Solution

What we clearly need is a relatively simple and convenient diet that enables immediate weight loss and long-term weight management without potential damage to our health. The Naturopathic Diet I have developed in my medical practice achieves these goals by training our body to use food as fuel rather than storing it as fat, leading to permanent weight loss and increasing our energy level. This is achieved with simple changes rather than with rigid dietary restrictions. There are two stages to the Naturopathic Diet: the weight loss stage, which adopts only the clinically proven elements of popular protein diets, and the weight maintenance stage, which restores a truly natural balance to the diet. Because our modern foods are often nutrient poor, this diet may need to be supplemented with vitamins, minerals, and herbs, which not only safely enhance weight loss, but also stabilize blood sugar and energy levels. And because our foods sources are often contaminated with toxins which not only threaten our health but impede weight loss, we need to choose 'clean' organic foods. The naturopathic diet not only leads to permanent weight loss but also detoxifies our bodies of disease causing toxins.

After years of eating a nutrient poor or imbalanced diet, our metabolism has been misled. We have, unknowingly, mimicked famine, teaching our bodies to secrete a high level of insulin following each meal. This promotes the storage of that food in preparation for a fast or famine. It prevents us from using that meal as an energy source and the body ultimately gains weight.

This process *is* reversible. We need to reverse it in order to lose weight and feel great. By re-educating the body and the hormonal (insulin) output following each meal, our original, more efficient metabolic state may be resumed.

Even when we have re-trained our metabolism this way, our diet still requires nutrient supplements. With growing emphasis on productivity and sales, the volume of food has increased but its nutrient value has diminished. Not only are many of the foods we eat grown on nutrient-poor soils, but they are also chemically encouraged to grow larger and more quickly. Just as a child cannot grow healthy and strong without proper nutrient intake, neither can our foodstuffs. The combination of nutrient-poor food and a busy lifestyle means we can no longer maintain an adequate intake of nutrients through food alone. We must supplement with vitamins and minerals in order to optimize the way our bodies function.

Re-educating our body through a properly balanced diet to use food as energy, not store it as fat, and supplementing our diet with an optimum level of nutrients and detoxifying our bodies of toxins – these are the fundamentals of naturopathic nutrition.

By 'naturopathic' nutrition, I mean a diet based on the principles of naturopathic medicine, especially the field of naturopathic medicine known as clinical nutrition. Naturopathic medicine combines the science of medicine with the art of lifestyle counseling to stimulate the body to heal itself and to support the patient during this process. The principles of naturopathic medicine are based on this goal:

First, do no harm
Co-operate with the healing powers of nature
Address the fundamental causes of disease
Heal the whole person through individualized treatment
Teach the principles of healthy living and preventative medicine

Prevention of disease is a central concept within naturopathic medicine. Patient education is an essential part of management for both treatment and prevention of illness. Naturopathic medicine indeed promotes education of the physical body itself, strengthening its component parts to improve overall health and resist disease. The underlying causative factors are identified and treated by natural methods, which also enhance our innate ability to heal.

Naturopathic medicine borrows from many ancient healing traditions. Naturopathic physicians are trained in the use of clinical nutrition, botanical or herbal medicine, homeopathic medicine, traditional Chinese medicine and acupuncture, hands-on techniques, and lifestyle counseling. Training for naturopathic medicine is extensive. A three year degree of pre-med study at university is followed by a four year, full-time program at a naturopathic college. In all licensed provinces or states, a naturopathic physician must also pass licensing exams (such as NPLEX in some states and provinces in North America) before being allowed to practice.

Nutrition or diet is the foundation of good health since the nutrients in our food are the building blocks of the body. We are what we eat, as the old saying goes. Clinical nutrition is the use of diet and nutrient supplements to prevent and treat diseases. Clinical nutrition has been practised for years and continues to grow in popularity. One of the forefathers of nutritional therapy was Linus Pauling, a renowned scientist and two-time Nobel Prize winner, whose books *Vitamin C and the Common Cold, Cancer and Vitamin C,* and *How To Live Better Longer* revolutionized our understanding of the role nutrients play in maintaining our health and treating disease conditions. His research and the work of his colleague and collaborator Dr Abram Hoffer, most notably in *Hoffer's Laws of Natural Nutrition,* continues to be supported by the complementary health community and reinforced by new research studies. For example, studies published in July of 2001 examined human blood levels of the ant-oxidant known as lutein (commonly found in dark green leafy vegetables) and its relationship to atherosclerosis. They found that those who ate diets rich in lutein had a 44% reduction in atherosclerotic lesions when compared to those who ate an "average" diet.

A naturopathic diet applies the science of clinical nutrition to the problem of losing excess weight and maintaining this loss before diet-based diseases like hypertension, diabetes, heart disease, and high cholesterol develop in our bodies; this diet is also effective in treating these disease conditions once they have developed. However, a naturopathic diet is more than the application of the science of clinical nutrition to weight loss and health; a naturopathic diet involves a lifestyle change in the way we eat, for the rest of our lives.

Since we are a society of convenience where time is scarce and the need for quick dietary solutions is valuable, recommendations for food preparation on this diet are customized for busy individuals, though some of the recipes are for some of us with the time to prepare more elaborate meals. The naturopathic program I have developed is an effective and safe for anyone who wishes to lose weight permanently. I have used this diet extensively in my practice and can assure you, it works!

Case Histories

In my practice as a naturopathic doctor at the Beresford Heart and Health Centre, I have prescribed the Naturopathic Diet for scores of patients wanting or needing to lose weight. The diet has been adapted and customized for each individual, but the results have been generally the same, regardless of the age, sex, or state of health.

Sam: 'Sam Jones' is a 32-year-old male who presented to my office complaining of fatigue and weight gain. He was concerned that he had gained 35 pounds over the previous 4 years without greatly changing his diet. Along with this weight gain, he experienced lethargy. Mid-afternoon would find him hungry and tired, craving a sweet or starchy food to help him through the rest of the workday. In addition to these symptoms, Sam reported a great deal of gas and bloating following each meal. He has a family history of adult onset diabetes and was concerned he may be developing early symptoms of this with his weight gain and fatigue.

After 8 weeks on the Naturopathic Diet, Sam had lost 23 pounds and reported little to no gas or bloating. His energy greatly increased after only 10 days on the diet, and his afternoon sweet cravings disappeared. Three years later, Sam has maintained a 37 pound weight loss and continues to use the Naturopathic Diet maintenance stage. He now reports having more energy, better concentration, and greater strength than before.

Pearl: 'Pearl Miner' is a 67-year-old female who presented with weight gain, high cholesterol, high blood pressure, and fatigue. She had tried several diets before coming to see me, all with very little success. She was discouraged with the weight gain following cessation of each diet she tried and was looking for a permanent solution.

Pearl's diet consisted mainly of starches, grains, fruits, and vegetables, with very little meat and fat. She thought that she was doing the "right thing" and could not understand why she continued to gain weight.

When she started the Naturopathic Diet, her initial weight was 187 pounds, with a waist measurement of 57 inches. After 10 days she had lost 6 pounds and 1.5 inches off her waist. Thrilled with her success and the simplicity of the diet, Pearl continued to lose 56 pounds and dropped to a 38 inch waist. The Naturopathic Diet has now become a lifestyle change for Pearl, who comments, "This was the easiest way to lose weight and keep if off. I will never go back to my old dietary habits again!"

John: 'John Law' is a 43-year-old male who reluctantly came to see me at the request of his medical doctor. A type II diabetic, his blood sugar levels had gradually increased over the past few years, as had his weight and blood pressure. In the preceding 6 months, he had required medications to help him control his blood sugars and blood pressure.

John initially weighed 245 pounds and had blood sugar levels that fluctuated between 7 mmol/l and 12 mmol/l. His blood pressure was 167/95. He was otherwise in good health and reported eating a diet rich in grains and fruits. He exercised 3 times a week.

After only 1 week on the Naturopathic Diet, his blood sugars had stabilized between 5 mmol/l and 7 mmol/l. He had lost 5 pounds and his blood pressure had decreased to 150/90. Eight weeks later John had lost 29 pounds and kept his blood sugar levels low. His blood pressure also remained between 118/78 and 127/84. He was told by his family physician that he no longer required any pharmacological aid to lower his blood pressure or blood sugar.

Since that time 1.5 years ago, he has lost 98 pounds and kept it off. More importantly, both his blood pressure and sugar levels remain within a healthy range.

Lawrence: 'Lawrence Tupper' is a 78-year-old male who presented with high cholesterol, high tryglycerides, high blood pressure, and excess body fat. He was already on lipitor to lower his cholesterol, but was told that he needed to lose weight in order to reduce further. Most medical doctors recommend that LDL cholesterol levels remain around 3.2, and will increase medication doses in order to achieve this. Lawrence took it upon himself to bring his levels down naturally and permanently. On 8 March, LT's blood lipids were as follows:

Total Cholesterol	7.7
LDL's	4.8
HDL's	1.2
Triglycerrides	1.7

At this time, his blood pressure was 172/87 and he weighed 234 pounds. His weight quickly dropped – by May 14 he weighed 214 pounds. His blood work was retested in August and November. In August, his total cholesterol was back down to normal at 4.45. He wanted to get it down further so that he could stop taking the Lipitor. By November he weighed 197 pounds and his blood pressure was 136/74. His blood work was as follows:

Total Cholesterol	3.66
LDL's	1.92
HDL's	1.37
Triglycerides	0.8

Lawrence has now integrated some of the restricted carbohydrates back into his diet and has not gained any weight back or increased his blood lipids levels.

Beyond these clinical cases, there are many others who have experienced positive results with the Naturopathic Diet, including several television talk show hosts and technicians on shows where I have been a guest.

Roberto Veri, host of Talk TV on the CTV network in Toronto, followed the Naturopathic Diet under my care, live on television for 10 weeks. During that time he lost 34 pounds and dropped 6%

of his body fat. Roberto never felt deprived and found the diet very easy to follow. As he remarked, "Penny's encyclopaedic knowledge and her attentiveness to her patients' concerns gives you a step-by-step foundation as to how your body works and how easy it is to comfortably slip into that healthy lifestyle you've always been meaning to get into."

Steve Ferris, a technician, enjoyed similar results. Steve first approached me complaining of symptoms associated with esophageal reflux. He was carrying around some extra weight that was increasing the intra-abdominal pressure and making digestion difficult. Along with herbal supplementation to help his stomach, Steve followed the Naturopathic Diet with great ease. Within a week he reported starting to feel much better. He has now made a lifestyle change, and although like everyone else on the diet, enjoys all food types, he maintains the healthy way of eating suggested in this book. He has never gained an ounce back. He comments, "I began the Naturopathic Diet due to extremely intense heart burn. Combined with too much weight and pressure around my stomach, I was not properly breaking down my food. Each time I ate I would be very nauseated and uncomfortable. I began the naturopathic diet to lose some weight and ease my stomach. When I started, I weighed 202 pounds. Three months later I had lost 31 pounds and never felt better. My stomach pain completely cleared. I have more energy than I had 15 years ago, and I gained a great deal of muscle. The Naturopathic Diet was easy to follow and I will always eat this way."

Glossary

Absorption: The selective taking-in or abstraction of water or other materials from the alimentary canal (digestive tract) into the blood or lymphatic system.

Acidosis: An accumulation of hydrogen in body fluids due to increased production as seen in a diabetic coma or failure of normal elimination by the kidney or excessive administration of acids.

Active Compound: A chemical agent that directly kills a pest. A constituent in a pesticide.

Adenosine Triphoshate (ATP): A compound containing three phosphates that when broken down produces energy and enables muscles and organs to function.

Adipose Tissue: The layer of fat found between the muscle and skin (subcutaneous), or around organs in the body.

Amino Acid: An inorganic nitrogen rich acid that forms the basic subunit of protein. Each subunit or amino acid is linked to another though a peptide bond. There are 8 essential amino acids (9 for infants) and 13 (or 12) non-essential acids for adults and children, respectively.

Anorexia: A condition of being without or having lost the appetite for food, leading to severe weight loss and associated with amenorrhea, the absence of menstruation, and psychological or physiological issues.

Anti-oxidant: A substance that neutralizes free radicals in the body. This aids the body in faster recover and promotes stronger, more healthy tissues.

Arteriosclerosis: A common blood vessel disorder characterized by calcified yellow plaques, lipids and debris that line the walls of the arteries.

Basal Metabolic Rate: The rate at which the body expends energy at rest for the maintenance activities such as organ function and breathing.

Bioavailability: The ability of ingested nutrients to pass through the digestive tract into and through the bloodstream to its destination cells.

Bioflavinoids: Also known as vitamin P, this group of plant pigments provide the colors to many plants and flowers. In humans they play a role in combating pain and inflammation, histamine, absorption of certain nutrients, and many other health benefits.

Biochemical Reactions: The chemical activities associated with life as exhibited in humans and other living organisms. These are the reactions that drive all bodily functions.

Biotin: A necessary vitamin for the body (also known as vitamin H), an essential co-factor in many enzymatic reactions.

Blood Pressure: The pressure of the blood measured against the walls of the arteries. Normal is considered 120/80.

Bovine Growth Hormone: Cow growth hormone, the hormone responsible for rapid growth and development of muscle size. This hormone is injected into cows to increase the rate of tissue growth and milk production.

Brown Fat: Fatty deposits found in particular places on the body such as between the shoulder blades. This is the type of fat that generates heat, particularly in hibernating animals.

Bulimia: Perpetual and voracious appetite for large quantities of food to a morbid degree. It is usually associated with vomiting the food after consumption and psychological issues.

Calcium: An essential mineral to the body necessary for bone strength, cardiac function, muscle regulation and much more.

Calorie: A unit that characterizes the amount of energy available from food.

Carbohydrate: An organic compound in nature consisting of carbon, hydrogen, and oxygen that is used by the body as a potential fuel source. This includes starches, sugars, fiber, cellulose, and gums.

Carnitine: An amine that is often considered an amino acid that helps to transport fat to the mitochondria to be burned for energy.

Cholecystokinin: A hormone formed in the presence of dietary fat that stimulates the contraction of the gall bladder and a sensation of fullness.

Cholesterol: A waxy substance present in all cell membranes that is important for the transportation and absorption of substances in and out of cells. Cholesterol is widely manufactured by the body and many dangers arise when it is produced in excess.

Chromium: An essential mineral for the body which helps to stabilize blood sugar levels.

Complex Carbohydrate: A carbohydrate that also contains fiber and has a slower release of sugar into the blood stream than a simple carbohydrate.

Coenzyme: A substance that must be present with an enzyme to allow that enzyme to function. Coenzymes are mandatory for the use of vitamins and minerals in the body.

Conjugated Linoleic Acid: An essential fatty acid.

Constipation: A condition in which stools are passed infrequently and with difficulty.

Detoxification: The process of ridding the body of poisonous chemicals, carcinogens, and other toxins.

Diarrhoea: The frequent passage of unformed liquid stools.

Diabetes: A disorder characterized by inadequate hormonal control of blood sugar levels associated with symptoms such as excessive urine excretion and thirst.

Diuretic: A substance that causes increased urine output by forcing the kidneys to excrete more salt, potassium, and water.

Edema: Fluid retention in the body resulting in swelling and bloating in the skin and other tissues.

Electrolytes: The ionized salts in the blood. A specific ratio known as the electrolyte balance is essential for proper bodily function.

Enzyme: One group of proteins produced in cells that are capable of greatly accelerating chemical reactions in the body without being broken down or consumed.

Essential Nutrients: Substances that the body cannot produce itself and are necessary for survival.

Extracellular: Outside the cell.

Fat Cell: A cell that stores fatty acids.

Fatty Acids: Components of fat molecules that can provide energy, but in high quantity can be harmful. These include cholesterol, triglycerides, prostaglandins, lecithin, choline, and others. There are essential fatty acids that the body cannot manufacture yet requires, and non-essential ones that it can make on its own.

Fiber: Plant compounds that are indigestible to the human digestive tract.

Free Radical: A highly reactive molecule that is known to injure cell membranes, damage DNA, and contribute to aging and degenerative illnesses.

Free Radical Scavenger: A substance like the anti-oxidant that seeks out and destroys free radicals in the body.

Free Range: The term used to describe farm animals that have access to the outdoors. This does not specify how much access and whether or not they have running space.

Fructose: A simple carbohydrate or sugar that comes from fruits and is absorbed and utilized by the body at a slower rate than glucose.

Garcinia Cambogia: A herb that helps to suppress appetite and prevents lipogenesis.

Genistein: An isoflavone found in soy products. (See Isoflavone)

Glucagon: A polypeptide hormone secreted by the pancreas in response to hypoglycemia. It is responsible for raising blood sugar levels when they fall too low.

Gluconeogenesis: The synthesis of glucose by the liver and kidneys from non-carbohydrate sources like amino acids and fatty acids.

Glucose: A simple carbohydrate or sugar, which is the end product of carbohydrate metabolism and is the main energy source for all living organisms.

Glutamine: An amino acid that has been shown to increase the rate of muscle growth in humans and decrease fat production.

Glycemic Index: A scale used to measure the availability of glucose present in different foods.

Glycogen: The main storage form of glucose, manufactured by and largely stored in the liver and muscles.

Glycogenolysis: The breakdown of glycogen stores in the liver to produce glucose in response to low blood sugar levels.

Growth Hormone: A polypeptide hormone secreted by the anterior pituitary gland. It acts on bone and muscle growth, and carbohydrate and nitrogen metabolism.

Guggulipids: A natural supplement that aids the liver in the breakdown and recycling of cholesterol as well as maximizing thyroid hormone output.

High-density Lipoproteins (HDL): Complexes of lipids and proteins that are important in structural and catalytic activities in cell membranes. These are the 'good' lipids that help prevent the 'bad' lipids (LDLs) from building up in the arteries.

Hormone: A chemical substance formed in one part of the body and transported to a different area where it has a regulatory effect on cellular function.

Hypercholesterolemia: An excess of cholesterol in the blood.

Hyperglycemia: An excessive amount of sugar in the blood.

Hyperinsulinemia: An excess of insulin secretion resulting in low blood sugar levels or hypoglycemia.

Hyperlipidemia: A condition in which lipids are present in excess in the blood.

Hypertension: Persistently high arterial blood pressure, usually diagnosed after three consecutive readings of 140/100 or more on three different dates.

Hypoglycemia: A low blood sugar concentration.

Inert Compound: A constituent in a pesticide that assists in the transport of the active compound and therefore does not directly kill the pest itself.

Insulin: A protein hormone formed and secreted by the pancreas in response to a rise in blood sugar level. It promotes lipid synthesis as it stores the sugar from the blood as fat.

Insulin-Like-Growth Factor 1: A hormone produced in the liver that controls cellular turnover, enhances fat breakdown, and increases energy. When abnormally high, it has been associated with an increase in cancer cell growth.

Insulin Resistance: A condition in which the body is insensitive or resistant to the effects of insulin. In most cases the body responds by producing even more insulin.

Isoflavone: A type of phytoestrogen found in soy products. (See Phytoestrogen)

Ketone Body: An acidic substance produced by the rapid metabolism of fatty acids.

Ketosis: The presence of excessive ketone bodies in the tissues, usually the result of starvation or diabetes mellitus.

Lipid: Fat or fatty substances including fatty acids, waxes, and steroids.

Lipogenesis: The formation of fat, and the transformation of non-fat materials into body fat.

Lipoprotein Lipase: An enzyme essential for the breakdown of fats to fatty acids and glycerol.

Liver: The central organ of metabolism of carbohydrates, proteins, and fats. It stores glycogen and takes part in regulating blood sugar levels and other essential substances such as vitamins and blood clotting factors. It is also the chief detoxifying organ of the body, rendering toxic or foreign substances innocuous.

Low Density Lipoproteins (LDL): Complexes of lipids and proteins found in the blood that contribute to heart disease and high cholesterol when produced in great concentrations.

Macronutrient: The nutrients that are required daily by the body in large amounts such as ounces and grams. They include protein, carbohydrates, lipids, and water.

Magnesium: An essential mineral for the body that plays a role in metabolism and muscle maintenance, and is required for many enzymatic reactions in the body.

Menopause: The cessation of spontaneous menstrual periods.

Metabolism: The chemical processes of every living cell in which energy is produced, tissues are built up (anabolism), and tissues are degraded (catabolism).

Micronutrient: Nutrients that are necessary in the diet in small amount, generally measured in milligrams or micrograms. They include vitamins, minerals, and herbs.

Mineral: An inorganic substance necessary for many structural and enzymatic roles in the body.

Mitochondria: The cell components that produce the energy required for metabolism. They are also called fat burners or power-house cells.

Naturopathy: Medical practice using natural substances and treatments such as diet, herbs, homeopathic remedies, and acupuncture to stimulate the body's innate healing response and produce therapeutic effects.

Neuropathy: A disease process characterized by the disintegration or destruction of specialized tissue in the nervous system. Resulting symptoms include numbness and tingling, pain, muscle weakness, and visual disturbances.

Obesity: An excessive accumulation of fat in the body, mainly deposited in the subcutaneous tissues. It is generally considered to be 30% above normal body weight.

Organic: The term used to describe both plants and animals that are farmed without pesticides, antibiotics, hormone injections, or genetically altered feed and are allowed to run in the open outdoors.

Organochlorines: A type of pesticide used on crops containing chlorine in its structure.

Organophosphates: A type of pesticide used on crops containing phosphate in its structure.

Pancreas: The organ or gland in the body which secretes insulin and glucagon upon differing metabolic demands to help regulate blood sugar levels.

Peroxides: Free radicals by-products produced when a molecule of fat reacts with oxygen in the body.

Pesticide: A chemical agent used to kill insects, fungus, or any other agent that may grow on or eat plants. This term includes herbicides, insecticides, and fungicides.

Phosphate: A mineral that is essential to the body for structure where it is exists in tissue, blood, bone, and in many chemical reactions.

Physiological: Pertaining to all the reactions and systems in the body and how they connect together to function as a whole.

Phytoestrogen: A type of phytosterol that mimics endogenous estrogen in the body. (See Phytosterol)

Phytosterol: A plant product with chemical properties similar to our own endogenous hormones.

Potassium: A mineral that is essential for the body and is found in high concentrations in tissues. It is necessary to maintain proper electrolyte balances in the body through its ionic charge and is used to excite or enhance action potential reactions.

Prostaglandins: A series of hormones, structurally similar to fatty acids, that are involved in cardiovascular and gastric functioning, inflammation, uterine contractions, etc.

Protein: A compound formed from nitrogen occurring in every living cell. It is essential for the growth, repair, and maintenance of every part of the body.

Psychology: The branch of science/medicine that deals with the mind and all mental processes.

RDA: Recommended Daily Allowance of vitamins, minerals, and other nutrients as suggested by the FDA (U.S.A. Food and Drug Administration).

Saturated Fats: A fatty acid that has every possible bond filled with hydrogen atoms and is therefore less reactive. They tend to be solid at room temperature and generally are from an animal origin.

Simple Carbohydrate: A simple form of sugar, such as glucose, lactose, or fructose, which is rapidly absorbed into the bloodstream. They are contained in foods such as pasta, potatoes, and candy.

Soy: A leguminous plant with many medicinal properties.

Starvation: A condition induced by continuous lack of sufficient food, causing renal failure, muscle cramping, and fatigue.

Thermogenesis: The production of heat or energy through an increase in metabolism above normal levels.

TOPO (DNA Topoisomerase): The enzyme involved in DNA replication, transcription, and differentiation.

Toxicity: An adverse, poisonous response that damages cells or alters chemical reactions in the body.

Triglyceride: A combination of glycerol and a fatty acid such as oleic or stearic acid. Most animal and vegetable fats are triglyceride esters and form the majority of ingested fat in the diet. High levels in the blood greatly increase the risk for heart disease.

Tyrosine Kinase: One enzyme that controls cell growth and differentiation.

Vasoconstriction: The narrowing of a blood vessel, which decreases blood flow and increases the pressure within it.

Vasodilation: The relaxation or expansion of a blood vessel, which increases blood flow and decreases blood pressure.

Vitamin: A constituent of the diet other than protein, carbohydrate, fat, and inorganic salts that is necessary for the growth and repair of the body.

Water Soluble: Ability to dissolve in water.

White Fat: The fat that is subcutaneous and found around the internal organs. This fat changes in size and is the fat lost during weight loss.

Diet & Nutrition

DIET & NUTRITION

What Is a Diet?

While the term 'diet' originally meant our usual food and drink, the word has assumed a new meaning in our society. No longer does it refer to an account of the nutritional habits of a population, but now has connotations of deprivation and starvation. No more is it related to growth, health, and energy, but rather to physical appearance. We go on a 'diet' to lose weight or to change our shape. Likewise, the once interchangeable term 'nutrition', which simply meant food or nourishment, has taken on new connotations, conjuring up images of energy-rich foodstuffs packed with essential vitamins and minerals.

In my opinion, diet and nutrition should be interchangeable terms which refer to the basic requirements needed by the human body to perform optimally. A diet is not a short-term solution to achieve a certain weight; it is a permanent pattern of eating. It is about learning to make the right food choices to maximize energy and output in order to maintain good health for the rest of our life.

Any dietary quick-fix that allows us to lose weight and then return to old dietary habits will never be successful. Choosing a diet is really a nutritional lifestyle choice. It establishes a lifelong pattern that shapes and forms health for the rest of our life. The right choice will produce the right shape!

What Is Food?

F ood is our body's potential energy, waiting to be converted into useable kinetic energy. The human body has several sources from which to manufacture energy. Ingested food is its number one preference. Following this we use the body's own fat stores, then finally its muscle.

Which energy source your body uses is up to us and is dictated by what foods we eat. At equilibrium, to maintain weight, we burn all the food we consume. To lose weight, we must stimulate the body to utilize our fat stores. This can be achieved given the right conditions.

All food is categorized into one of three groups:

Fats

Carbohydrates

Proteins

Each affect the body by directing it towards a different biochemical pathway. It is important to understand the difference between these food groups in order to comprehend which foods encourage fat storage, and which stimulate its breakdown. Although it is rare that any one food contains only fat or carbohydrate or protein alone, certain foods may be predominantly of one type and therefore act metabolically like that food group.

What Is Fat?

Fat is also known as lipid. Two main groups of fats exist, and they are differentiated by the number of hydrogen bonds between each link in the fat compound. A 'saturated fat' is one that has all possible bonds filled up with hydrogen. It is therefore saturated with hydrogen and is considered solid in nature. This type is found in animal fat. Due to the fact that saturated fats contain completely filled bonds, they are quite stable with no free bonds for the body to interact with. 'Unsaturated fats' are less stable because not all their bonds are filled with hydrogen. Thus the empty bonds leave spaces that have the potential to react with other atoms or substances in the body.

It is important to recognize that not all fats are bad and that we do need some fat in the diet, especially unsaturated fats.

The role of saturated fats, or their breakdown unit, fatty acid, is extremely limited. They only serve as calories. Since they cannot interact with the body, they cannot aid in any bodily function. However, unsaturated fats, especially 'essential' fatty acids, play a large role in the body. These fats are involved in the production of prostaglandins, cell membrane construction, hormone regulation, and many other body systems.

Fat sends a signal of satisfaction to the brain upon ingestion via the production of a hormone called CCK or cholecystokinin. Without this hormone, we continue to eat, our body waiting for the satiety signal. People on fat-free diets continually feel unsatisfied as they never receive the CCK hormonal message. They keep on eating to try and achieve this feeling, even though they are not nutritionally deprived.

Within the body there are two types of fat deposition. Brown fat, which is quite scarce and decreases in concentration as we age, exists only in certain areas of the body like the back of the neck and between the shoulder blades. We cannot produce more brown fat in our lifetime. Its main purpose is to generate heat through redundant metabolic cycling, a process by which calories are burned without producing any useable substances. This process is essential in infancy and childhood but becomes less important with maturity.

Most of the fat on the body is white fat, which is deposited subcutaneously (under the skin), in the abdomen or around the internal organs. This is the fat that changes in concentration throughout life – and this is the type of fat we are talking about losing. Of interest, the production of new fat cells only occurs during the first few years of life. It is theorized that overfeeding children results in the production of excess numbers of fat cells which then remain with us for life. By the time we reach puberty, the number of fat cells in our body is fixed. We can neither increase nor decrease their number (unless under the care of a surgeon!). However, the *amount* of fat they contain can vary tremendously, and this is the way in which we lose or put on fatty weight.

What Is Carbohydrate?

Carbohydrates, unlike essential fatty acids, vitamins, minerals, or protein, are not considered building blocks for the body, but are short-term energy sources. Their break-down product is a sugar called glucose. To use carbohydrates as fuel rather than storing them as fat, we must follow certain guidelines, such as ingesting specific amounts at certain times and selecting particular types of carbohydrates.

There are two main types of carbohydrates, simple and complex. Simple carbohydrates, like bread and pastry flours, contain only sugars and starches. The simple carbohydrates are broken down very quickly as they have weak chemical bonds and will therefore raise blood sugar levels rapidly following ingestion.

Complex carbohydrates like fresh fruits and vegetables are a combination of fiber with or without sugar and starch. Fiber cannot be broken down and therefore cannot contribute to increased glucose levels in the blood. This explains why complex carbohydrates that are high in fiber only contain one-third the amount of calories found in fat and simple carbohydrates. As well, complex carbohydrates provide the fiber that helps keep the digestive tract clean. Fiber promotes rapid transit through the bowel and binds toxins which are subsequently expelled in the stools. Not all complex carbohydrates are low in starch or sugar, even though they contain fiber, so careful decision making as to which carbohydrates we eat is very important.

What Is Protein?

Protein is the basic building block of the body, the single most important nutrient. Protein is used for the growth of every cell in the body. Our brain cells, enzymes, many hormones, antibodies, muscle, and even blood cells are made of protein. Discounting water, over half the body weight of an average individual is protein. This protein is continually being broken down and replaced. Studies show that over 90% of the body has completely turned over within one year. This process requires nutritional protein.

When digested, protein is broken down into smaller subunits called amino acids. There are 29 amino acids that form hundreds of different proteins in the body. The liver is capable of producing approximately 80% of the amino acids that we need. These amino acids are therefore considered non-essential to the diet. The other 20%, however, cannot be manufactured by the body and must be obtained from our diet.

Not only is protein an important stimulus for weight loss, it is essential for the integral maintenance of the body. It is easy to comprehend how a deficiency of protein can result in serious malfunction in any number of systems. Poor immunity, muscle fatigue, slow tissue healing, and dry skin and hair are just a few examples of protein deficiency.

What Happens When We Eat?

The breakdown and absorption of food in our body varies according to the type of food we ingest. Digestion is accomplished largely by enzymes that break down food into smaller components that can pass through the lining of the gut into the bloodstream.

Digesting Fats

Among the food groups, the digestion of fat is the most complicated. Fat tends to aggregate in large sheets. The first part of fat breakdown, therefore, becomes digesting the large lipid sheets into small droplets to increase the surface area over which the appropriate enzymes can work. This is achieved through bile salts, which act in a similar manner to detergent on grease. This process is called emulsification. Once emulsified, the lipase enzymes secreted by the pancreas are free to break down the fatty acid bonds. The broken down fat units, mixed with bile and cholesterol, form units called micelles. The combination of micelles and other lipid digestion products results in an environment suitable for fat uptake by the intestinal cells. Once absorbed, the fat breakdown molecules (fatty acids, glycerol, cholesterol, and lysolecethin) are re-packaged as droplets called chylomicrons that are released into the lymphatic system and from there reach the blood.

Fats and Disease

Some fats are required for health while others can be harmful. Whether a fat benefits or harms the body depends on several factors, not only the type of fat (saturated or unsaturated) but also the temperature of the fat, its age, its exposure to other substances like oxygen and light, and how much we eat.

A saturated fat tends to be much less chemically stable and is therefore quite susceptible to reaction with light and oxygen. This creates free radicals within the body, which in turn attack cells and the lining of arteries, creating inflammation and degeneration. A diet rich in saturated fats has been shown to increase the rate of many diseases, most notably cardiovascular disease. In general, free radicals attack a cell in one of two ways. First, they can damage the DNA of a cell to the point of cell death. This is actually the better of the two scenarios as the cell simply dies and the body ages more quickly. However, if the free radical mutates the cell and then alters its replication pattern, it can increase the risk of cancer in the body. As saturated fats are more susceptible to free radicalization than any other nutrient in the body, it only makes sense to lower them in our diet.

Most people consume too much fat in the diet. Each gram of fat contains more than twice the number of calories as a gram of carbohydrate or protein. Any lipid or fat that is not immediately used by the body for energy or structures such as cell membranes is immediately put into storage. It is easy to see then why a diet rich in fat can easily increase weight.

There is another side of the coin, though. We actually do need some fat. The good or essential fats, such as omega 3, 6, and 9 found in fish oils and flax seeds, for example, are important for many different functions in the body, such as the transfer of oxygen from the lungs to the blood, cell membrane structure, proper brain function, proper nerve transmission, efficient wound healing, healthy skin, and more. A diet that is deficient in good fats can impair function and weaken tissue structure.

Dietary fat does not affect our blood cholesterol and fat levels as much as we may think. Essential fatty acids actually lower the levels of these blood lipids and are thus beneficial. Dietary saturated fats are responsible for about 20% of your blood cholesterol, the remaining 80% is due to the combination of high insulin and carbohydrates.

Fat Facts

✦ Saturated fats increase free radical formation
✦ Free radicals cause tissue damage and increase cancer risk
✦ Some essential fats are needed in the diet and lower cholesterol
✦ High blood cholesterol levels are mostly due to carbohydrates in association with high insulin

Digesting Carbohydrates

Carbohydrate digestion begins in the mouth where amylase, an enzyme secreted by the salivary glands, begins to break the bonds between the glucose molecules. This enzyme can only breakdown polysaccharides (multiple bonded glucose units) into smaller units, not into single glucose molecules. The final carbohydrate digestion takes place in the intestinal tract by enzymes on the wall cell surface. Finally, glucose is moved across the wall by a specific ion pump and into the blood for use.

Energy Sources

The sugars found in carbohydrates are the principal source of energy for the body, and the principal sugars found in carbohydrates are glucose and fructose. Both glucose and fructose are monosaccharides or single sugar units that are metabolized to form ATP (Adenosine Triphosphate), the body's energy source. While fructose is mainly found in honey and fruit, glucose is extremely abundant in many foods and serves as the building block of most carbohydrates. Glucose is also the sugar found in the blood stream; the body uses blood as its glucose delivery system to feed the tissues. Extra glucose is stored in the liver and muscles in a form called glycogen. When in excess, glucose is stored in adipose tissue as fat.

The chart below shows the availability of our different sources of energy. Phosphagen and muscle glycogen are anaerobic sources, requiring no oxygen. The others – glucose, fatty acids, and amino acids – are aerobic, requiring oxygen. The chart lists the source, the materials used and produced, and the amount of energy produced per molecule. The last column indicates how long it takes for the body to use up each source.

Sources of Energy

Type	Substrate (material used)	Product (material produced)	Energy M ATP	Time
Phosphagen	Phosphocreatine	Creatine+PO3	1	8-10 secs
Muscle Glycogen	Glucose	Lactic acid	2.5	1.3-6.3 mins
Aerobic	Fatty Acids | + O2	CO2 + H2O	4	unlimited
	Amino Acids |			

In an average individual about 400 mg of glycogen is stored in skeletal muscle and provides a fuel reserve of glucose. This only lasts 1.3-6.3 minutes. (The 100 mg of glycogen found in the liver is a backup supply of glucose to maintain blood levels during fasting.) Beyond 6 minutes, energy is obtained from the aerobic metabolism of fatty acids, amino acids, and newly synthesised glucose. Phosphocreatine is stored in muscle and is readily available to initiate contraction. However, it is extremely limited and is used up in a few seconds.

There are two important features of this chart that relate directly to the discussion of a good diet:

1. The amount of stored glycogen is limited to the small amounts noted above (except in a few, rare genetic disorders). Most of the time, the stores are full, and even after exercise, it only takes a small amount of dietary sugar to replenish them. Once full, excess carbohydrate is re-routed, converted into fat, and stored as adipose tissue.

2. The aerobic sources which provide the majority of our energy are fatty acids and amino acids. Insulin promotes fat storage and limits our access to fat as a source of energy. Although insulin normally promotes protein synthesis, there is evidence that at chronically high levels (such as is seen in hyperinsulinaemia) protein synthesis is inhibited and muscle breakdown may occur to provide amino acids for glucose production. The Naturopathic Diet aims to reverse our high insulin levels, promoting use of fatty acids and the breakdown of our fat stores while preserving muscle.

Blood Sugar Levels

Sugar levels increase quickly after a high carbohydrate meal and slowly return to normal as the glucose is utilized. However, blood glucose levels must remain at a fairly constant level for the body to function properly. There are a myriad of hormones involved in regulating blood sugar levels, but we are only going to concern ourselves with two, insulin and glucagon (not to be confused with glycogen, the storage form of glucose).

Insulin is produced in the beta cells of the pancreas. Sometimes referred to as the 'feasting' hormone or the 'storage' hormone, insulin is released when blood sugar levels rise, and works by increasing the uptake of glucose from the blood and storing this sugar as glycogen and then fat. Glucagon is a hormone secreted from the alpha cells of the pancreas when blood sugar levels fall too low. It has an opposite effect to that of insulin. Glucagon functions in two major ways. First, it causes the breakdown of glycogen stored in the liver, a process is known as glycogenolysis. Second, glucagon initiates gluconeogenesis in the liver, the formation of glucose from other molecules such as amino acids, glycerol (from fats), lactate, and pyruvate. These two processes together promote the release of glucose into the blood to help raise sugar levels back to normal.

Insulin and glucagon thus work in tandem to help keep blood sugar levels within a narrow range. Continual abuse or stress upon this system through large swings in sugar levels from increased amounts of carbohydrate can produce an insensitivity reaction whereby more hormone is required to produce the same response, a response akin to drug addiction where higher concentrations of a drug may be needed to elicit the same reaction. This response takes many years of 'carbohydrate abuse' to develop, but when it does, we get into trouble not only with our weight but also with our health.

The Hypoglycemia-Hyperglycemia Connection

Hypoglycemia is a condition in which blood glucose levels are abnormally low. This often occurs in reaction to hyperglycemia or high sugar levels following a high carbohydrate meal. After the ingestion of carbohydrates the breakdown of food into sugar is quite rapid. This sugar is then delivered to the blood and glucose levels rise. The faster the breakdown of food into sugar, the faster the delivery of sugar, and the higher the blood sugar levels rise. Due to the fact that the simple building blocks of carbohydrates are sugars and the bonds between them are weak relative to that of protein, a large amount of glucose is formed and delivered quickly to the blood after a meal rich in carbohydrates. It is here that insulin is called upon to scoop up all this sugar and carry it out of the blood. Glycogen stores are full and it is therefore deposited as fat.

A few hours later, most of this meal has been stored as fat and our blood sugar levels are now too low, hypoglycemia. Our body senses this and we feel very tired, dizzy, and possibly nauseated. Then our body begins to crave foods that will release sugar into the blood quickly, such as a sweets or a starch. It is a rare individual who craves a piece of chicken when they are hypoglycemic! Most of us indulge in carbohydrates, once again raising our blood-sugar levels and starting the whole process anew.

If you find that by 10:00 a.m. or 3:00 p.m. you are tired and hungry, take a look at your diet. Your breakfast or lunch was probably high in carbohydrates, creating this problem.

Carbohydrate Facts:

When we eat a high carbohydrate meal:
* Hyperglycemia (high blood sugar level) is induced
* Insulin is secreted, hypoglycemia (low sugar) results, and food is stored as fat
* Carbohydrates are craved and then ingested
* The cycle goes round again

Insulin Resistance

Most North Americans have grown up on a diet that is high in carbohydrates. Cereal or toast for breakfast, a sandwich for lunch and pasta for dinner. Over the years our insulin-glucagon system has been over-worked to the point of insensitivity. Our hormone responses have become exaggerated in order to achieve the same effect. Approximately three out of four Americans have a slight to serious problem with their blood sugar level control mechanisms. This is known as insulin resistance, where there is a decreased reaction to insulin output, thereby stimulating extra insulin release. This extra insulin in our blood (hyperinsulinemia) acts as a barrier to using the existing fat in our bodies by blocking access to it.

If we need glucose or energy and cannot access our fat, we must look to alternate sources. Muscle is where our body turns, and slowly we eat away at our lean body tissue mass. Inside the muscle are mitochondria, the fat burning units, which are subsequently lost, thereby decreasing our potential to lose weight. For these reasons, it becomes clear that through a high carbohydrate diet it is almost impossible to lose weight while remaining in this biochemically undesirable state.

More Carbohydrate Facts:

✦ High carbohydrate diets lead to insulin resistance
✦ High levels of insulin block fat usage
✦ Inability to use fat results in muscle breakdown and less weight loss
✦ Weight is perpetually gained

Carbohydrates and Disease

Hypoglycemia and excess weight gain, although not very desirable, are not life threatening. However, left untreated, these relatively minor conditions may develop into very serious diseases. These diseases are simply extensions of hyperinsulinemia.

Food related diseases have been on the rise for centuries. In ancient Egypt, the farming of grains fostered a high-carbohydrate, low-fat diet, and heralded the appearance of food related diseases. Their diet was very similar to ours today and so were their diseases: mummification records show evidence of obesity, high blood pressure, high cholesterol, and heart disease.

High Cholesterol

Hypercholesterolemia is the term used to define high cholesterol levels in the blood. This is a large contributing factor towards heart disease as cholesterol is primarily responsible for the blockages that occlude the vessels supplying the heart muscle. Hypercholesterolemia continues to affect a high percentage of the population, despite the trend toward low-fat products over the past few decades. The reason for this is that what we eat only accounts for 18% of our blood lipid levels. A high fat diet will increase cholesterol levels, but only very slightly. The same holds true for decreasing cholesterol with a low-fat diet. The remaining 82% is manufactured by our liver irrespective of our dietary fat intake. It is insulin that commands the liver to increase the production of cholesterol. It is those carbohydrates, even those that are fat free and cholesterol free, that are increasing our cholesterol level. Sitting on our dinner table they appear to be the ideal food type for one with high cholesterol, but as soon as they are ingested, it is a completely different story. We need to work on lowering our cholesterol by manipulating the 82% in our blood levels derived from carbohydrates more so than the 18% derived from fats.

Cholesterol Facts:

+ Dietary cholesterol accounts for only 18% of the blood cholesterol level
+ The liver produces 82% of blood cholesterol
+ Insulin instructs the liver to produce more cholesterol
+ Therefore carbohydrates increase cholesterol at a higher rate than those foods that are high in protein with a little cholesterol in them

Hypertension

Hypertension is another disease that afflicts a high proportion of the population. Hypertension is defined as an increase in blood pressure above 140 (systolic)/100(diastolic), where normal blood pressure is 120/80. A rise in blood pressure is usually the result of one or both of the following:

1. An increase in total fluid within the blood vessels. Basically, if you increase the volume within a closed container, then the pressure inside increases.
2. Narrowing of the blood vessels. It requires more pressure to force the blood through tighter tubes.

Insulin can potentially increase blood pressure through both mechanisms listed above. When insulin is in excess, it directs the kidneys to retain more salt. When the body retains salt, it will always retain extra water so that the electrolyte balance in the body remains somewhat constant. This excess fluid will not only cause bloating and discomfort but will raise our blood pressure significantly. Thus a decrease in insulin allows the kidneys to release the salt, and therefore the water, ultimately lowering blood pressure.

Insulin also appears to influence arterial wall thickness and the development of atherosclerosis (hardening of the arteries). Narrower arteries lead to increased blood pressure.

Hypertension Facts:

❋ Insulin stimulates the kidneys to retain salt
❋ Extra salt means excess fluid retention
❋ Insulin can influence vessel diameter
❋ Increased fluids and vessel narrowing result in high blood pressure levels

Heart Disease

Not only is high cholesterol a contributing factor towards heart disease, but so are high triglycerides. Triglycerides are another type of fat in the blood, and they create problems for the heart. Insulin is the culprit here, too.

High insulin levels have been shown to result in thickening of the arteries, more extensive and complex plaque development, and increased thrombosis, all of which increase the risk of cardiovascular disease. High glucose and insulin levels are known to alter sorbitol metabolism within the arterial walls, and it may be this that results in thickening and plaque formation. Diabetics with chronically high glucose levels develop more extensive vascular damage than individuals with similar cholesterol/triglyceride levels and no diabetes. Studies have shown artery thickness to be increased in subjects with hyperinsulinemia.

Heart Disease Facts:

❖ Insulin increases production of cholesterol and triglycerides
❖ High insulin and glucose result in thickening of arteries, vessel damage, and thrombosis
❖ Vessel damage and higher blood lipids significantly increase the risk of heart disease

---

Diabetes

Diabetes mellitus is a disorder of carbohydrate metabolism characterized by higher than normal blood sugar levels (hyperglycemia). This results both from an impaired insulin response to glucose and, in Type II diabetics, from decreased insulin effectiveness at the tissue level (insulin resistance). Most Type II patients retain some insulin secretion, but the response to glucose is severely decreased.

Diabetes mellitus is divided into two types: Type-I or insulin-dependant, and Type-II, non-insulin dependant. Type-I accounts for 15-20% of all cases, and individuals must inject extra insulin to help lower blood sugar levels. Type-II individuals retain some insulin secretion but often need oral medication to augment it.

Diabetes	Type-I	Type-II
Age of Onset	< 30 years	> 30 years
Insulin secretion	Almost absent	Delayed and reduced
Insulin resistance	No	Frequent
Diet causally related	No	Yes
Require insulin	Yes	Not initially
Response to oral medication	None	Good
Associated Conditions (Retinopathy, neuropathy vascular disease, nephropathy etc.)	Yes	Yes

Type-II diabetes results from persistently high blood sugars in susceptible individuals. Chronic hyperglycemia has an almost toxic effect on the beta cells of the pancreas. This leads to a delayed and decreased insulin secretion in response to high blood glucose. This toxic effect can often be reversed and insulin secretion returned to normal by prolonged stabilization of blood sugar levels with diet and weight loss.

Diabetes Facts:

✦ Hyperglycemia leads to increased insulin secretion
✦ Constant hyperglycemia decreases insulin sensitivity to glucose
✦ Insulin resistance results in uncontrolled high blood sugar
✦ High blood sugars promote weight gain
and diabetes-related disorders

Digesting Protein

Protein digestion begins in the stomach with the aid of proteases. Proteases are enzymes secreted in the stomach that break the bonds in amino acid chains. Once again, only 15% of these bonds are broken down in the stomach. The other 85% are hydrolyzed in the intestinal wall by the brush-border (cell wall) enzymes. The single amino acids are then transported out of the gastro-intestinal tract and into the plasma for use.

Proteins are large molecules made up of single amino acids linked together. Most amino acids can take on one of two forms. The different forms are mirror images of each other. The different forms are called L- and D-series. Due to the fact that the L-series of amino acids are structurally the same as those found in plants and animal tissues, they are biochemically the form the choice. When we speak of dietary protein, both the order and the ratio of the amino acids it contains is important. In order for a protein to be complete, it must contain all 29 different amino acids. By changing the order of the amino acids in a protein, we can form more that 70,000 different proteins and enzymes. Each different type of protein therefore has its own signature series of amino acids that allows us to identify it from other proteins.

Of the approximately 29 different amino acids, the liver produces about 80% of these from different dietary sources such as incomplete proteins. These are called *non-essential* amino acids. However, approximately 20% of amino acids cannot be manufactured and must be ingested directly. These are the *essential* amino acids.

Amino acids also contain nitrogen. This is one of the major distinguishing factors of protein from carbohydrates and fats in the body. We use this level of nitrogen to determine the protein's biological value. A protein that is high in nitrogen, like an egg, will have a high biological value. The higher the biological value of a protein, the more readily it is digested. As nitrogen is excreted from the body, the value of a protein then becomes a ratio between the incoming nitrogen levels versus the excreted levels. When there is a positive balance, there is extra protein or substrate to go into tissue growth, hormones, and antibody production. When the nitrogen balance is negative, our body will begin to degrade our muscle in order to provide the amino acids necessary for the function of the body.

Protein and Disease

The production and degradation of proteins from amino acids in the body is a continuous process. When our body requires more enzymes or hormones or begins tissue repair, more protein needs to be produced. If we do not maintain an adequate dietary intake during these periods, we begin to break down muscle to replace the deficit.

Not only will a diet deficient in protein weaken the body and make it vulnerable to disease, it will also increase the rate of weight gain. The hormonal changes induced by a protein-deficient diet will teach the body to store our food as fat and hold our fat stores. Protein has a profound effect on the control of insulin secretion. As we have seen, when insulin rises after a meal rich in carbohydrates, not only does the food, now in the form of blood glucose, become stored as fat and therefore is not used as a fuel source, that rise in insulin itself has a variety of other adverse effects. Insulin directs the liver to produce cholesterol and triglycerides. It interacts with our blood vessels, encouraging them to thicken and constrict, thus raising blood pressure. This increase in blood pressure is then augmented by the effect of insulin on the kidneys, where it instructs them to hold onto salt and subsequently water. Finally, continued high secretion of insulin in response to high blood sugar levels leads to insulin resistance.

Protein moderates post-prandial hyperglycaemia and thus reduces insulin secretion. Protein, therefore, is not only beneficial in terms of tissue repair and metabolic function, it is also crucial in the reversal of hyperinsulinaemia and its attendant diseases.

Protein Facts:

✦ Protein is the most essential nutrient
✦ Protein provides the building material for most tissue and reactions in the body
✦ The type of protein is important – complete vs. incomplete
✦ Protein deficiency weakens the body and promotes weight gain

---

Lowering Body Fat

The message our body has received from a high-carbohydrate diet is to store food as fat, thanks to insulin resistance and high blood levels of glucose. To reverse this process, burn our fat, and use our food as energy, we must reduce the dramatic rise in blood sugar levels that occurs with each meal. Then there will be no stimulus for high insulin secretion. Once insulin is lowered, the sugar in our blood following a meal will slowly be dispersed to the brain, muscles, and other areas of the body that require energy. Once this fuel source is depleted, the body requires an alternative source of energy. Fat is an ideal substrate. Our metabolism is now free to break apart existing fat cells, releasing energy-dense fats to replenish the blood. This is possible because insulin is no longer blocking the use of the fat or adipose tissue. Similarly, the use of fat as an energy source in the powerhouse mitochondria of muscle cells is facilitated.

A diet high in protein but low in carbohydrates will enable our body to do this. The glycemic index of protein is low and will not raise blood sugar levels following ingestion. In addition, protein acts to slow the release of sugars from simultaneously ingested carbohydrates into the blood. Following a high protein meal there is no longer a massive rush of sugar into blood, spiking glucose levels. Instead, there is a nice even flow of sugar that lasts much longer, creating a full or satisfied feeling that carries us from meal to meal. Without a spike in glucose, there is no excess release of insulin and therefore no fat storage.

Dramatic reductions in triglyerides are also seen by following a high-protein, low-carbohydrate diet. By lowering insulin and glucose we not only lower our blood lipid levels but also repair and increase the integrity of the vessels themselves.

Protein also helps preserve lean body mass such as muscle. Protein combined with exercise helps to build more muscle. By preserving muscle, we are maintaining the use of our mitochondria – our fat burners – and once again increasing the rate of weight loss.

More Protein Facts:

➤ Protein results in lower blood sugar levels

➤ Protein reduces insulin release, decreases fat storage
and increases fat breakdown

➤ Protein preserves and promotes muscle growth

The Naturopathic Diet Program

Stage One: The Weight Loss Stage
Protein Portions
Good Protein Food Sources
Carbohydrates and Glycemic Indices
Good and Bad Carbohydrate Food Sources
Unlimited Vegetables
Limited Vegetables and Legumes
Restricted Vegetables
Fruits
Other Limited Carbohydrates
Forbidden Carbohydrates
Condiments
Beverages

Stage Two: The Weight Maintenance Stage
Reintroduction Order

Rate of Weight Loss

Health Benefits and Positive Side Effects
Weight Loss
Improved Digestion
Lowered Insulin Levels
Detoxification
Prevention and Treatment of Disease

Safety

THE NATUROPATHIC
DIET PROGRAM

Rising blood sugar levels stimulate the release of insulin, which ultimately stores the food we eat as fat. This is the factor that has contributed to our society's weight problem; this is the factor we must reverse through our diet.

If we had maintained a balanced diet from childhood, we would not be trapped in the current nutritional crisis. Our bodies would not have developed insulin resistance and its attendant problems. Our goal is to retrain our bodies to a biochemical state similar to that of childhood. Once this is achieved, we can again enjoy a variety of different foods without gaining weight. To sustain this renewed metabolism and not undo or reverse the changes, balanced meals are still recommended.

All this can be done through the Naturopathic Diet.

This is not a diet change that we make temporarily until we lose the weight that we wish to lose and then return to the bad eating habits we had before. Any diet change that is not a lifestyle change only results in temporary weight loss. There is no need to restrict ourselves completely from all the foods we love, however. By making a few additions to our diet (instead of restrictions), we will be able to eat almost anything we wish after the initial weight-loss period. We can return to a variety of different foods without any fear of regaining the weight.

The Naturopathic Diet progresses in two main stages. The *first stage* is the weight loss stage, lasting about eight weeks. The diet here is protein rich and slightly carbohydrate restricted, especially simple carbohydrates. The *second stage* is the maintenance stage. Part of the maintenance diet is the continued inclusion of protein at each meal, but here the dietary choices expand, allowing us freedom to enjoy many different types of food. Weight loss ends but no weight is gained. If we return to a diet of high carbohydrates and low protein, we will undo all the metabolic changes that were brought about by the Naturopathic Diet.

Stage One: The Weight Loss Stage

The weight loss stage of the Naturopathic Diet involves a limited period of time, for two good reasons. First, the diet 'retrains' the body's metabolism in eight to nine weeks as a rule. During these weeks, blood sugar, and thus insulin levels, remain consistently low. During this time, the body learns the connection between protein and low glucose. The message it receives each time protein is ingested is that the blood sugar levels are low so it does not need to secrete insulin at a high rate. Once the body has practiced and consolidated this message for a period of time, we can then combine some higher glycemic-index carbohydrates with our protein and the insulin secretion will remain low. This is what we do in stage two. Protein will always act as a cue, keeping the insulin release small and maintaining the weight loss. This is good, as we do not have to remain on such a rigid diet forever!

The second reason for limiting the time period of this stage is that we do not wish to keep losing weight forever! At the end of the eight to nine week period, however, if we *do* wish to lose more weight, we simply continue with stage one of the diet until the desired loss is achieved. This is a very nutrient-rich diet that may be followed for long periods of time without adversely affecting your health. The foods recommended all contain high quantities of vitamins, minerals, and protein, of course. These same foods are very low in 'empty calories' – calorie-dense foods that have little nutritional value. There is essentially no limit to the length of time we may stay in stage one. However, we most likely will stop losing weight once excess fat has been eradicated.

If we *are* ready to stop losing weight after this initial eight to nine week period, then we can simply move into stage two, the maintenance stage. This is where we will remain for the rest of our life.

Protein Portions (Stage One)

The exact amount of protein each individual requires varies from person to person, depending on a number of different factors, including sex, size, and energy demands, but within the general population there is an average range of protein intake that can be applied, ranging from 15 to 30 grams. A smaller female should use the numbers at the lower end of the food-gram ranges, a larger male, the high end of the scale.

Regardless of sex or body size, each meal must contain 15 to 25 grams (0.5-1 ounces) of protein. The body requires this amount to signal the lowered insulin reaction. We may eat slightly more than this amount or we may snack on protein between meals, but we cannot go under this range. If we do, the body will not receive an adequate message – and our blood sugar levels will not remain stable and low.

So how much is 15 to 25 grams? We don't need to weigh our food or count our grams – just compare it to the size of our hand. The average hand is approximately 16 cm or 6 inches long. We only need a piece of protein around 10-11 cm or 4 inches long and 2 cm or 3/4 inch thick. Thus about 3/4 the size of your hand per meal. Again, we can increase this amount slightly or snack on protein between meals, but we cannot decrease it.

Where do we start? We need to start each day with a power protein breakfast to stimulate our body and our metabolism into action. We cannot skip breakfast or any other meal, for that matter. If we do, we will put your body into starvation mode, and it will store whatever food it receives next, irrespective of what it is. Breakfast is particularly important. We have already fasted overnight, and this is the cycle we need to break to jump-start our metabolism in the morning. This meal sets a precedent for the rest of the day, both physiologically and psychologically. If we skip breakfast, or only eat carbohydrates, our body will feel very tired and our metabolism will slow. This in turn may depress us, at which point we are more likely to eat the wrong things again as our body will crave sugar to raise our depleted blood glucose levels. We don't want to start the day in that cycle.

Good Protein Food Sources

Protein is required each meal. In order to determine the amount of protein in various food source portions, we can refer to the first table presented here. This table shows how much of each protein food source we must eat in order to obtain a certain amount of dietary protein. For example, a chicken breast measuring about the size of our hand (about 115 grams or 4 ounces) contains about 30 grams of protein. The remaining weight is made up of water, fat, and carbohydrate. The table lists the required intake to obtain two different protein portions, for the small female and the large male. Measurements are listed in terms of weight and food quantity or cups to make the information easier to follow.

The second table allows us to refine our protein choices. We do not want to consume high-fat protein sources very frequently. This table lists the ratio of protein to fat in each protein type and therefore makes it easier to choose low-fat protein sources to increase our weight loss and to improve the diet's health benefits.

Dietary Protein Content of Common Food Sources

Food Source	Diet Requirement 15-20 grams (0.5-0.7 ounces)	Diet Requirement 20-30 grams (0.7-1.1 ounces)
Eggs	3 whites and 2 yolks	5 whites and 3 yolks
Tofu (extra firm/low fat)	84-112 g (3-4 oz.)	140-168 g (5-6 oz.)
Beef (lean)	70-84 g (2.5-3 oz.)	98-112 g (3.5-4 oz.)
Veal	70-84 g (2.5-3 oz.)	98-112g (3.5-4 oz.)
Pork	56-84 g (2-3 oz.)	84-112 g (3-4 oz.)
Chicken	70-84 g (2.5-3 oz.)	98-112 g (3.5-4 oz.)
Turkey	70-84 g (2.5-3 oz.)	98-112 g (3.5-4 oz.)

Cottage Cheese (low fat)	3/4 cup	1 cup
Ricotta Cheese (low fat)	3/4 cup	1 cup
Salmon	70-98 g (2.5-3.5 oz.)	98-126 g (3.5-4.5 oz.)
Tuna	70-98 g (2.5-3.5 oz)	98-126 g (3.5-4.5 oz.)
Trout	70-98g (2.5-3.5 oz.)	98-126 g (3.5-4.5 oz.)
Protein Powder	dependant on make	dependant on make
Protein Bar	dependant on make	dependant on make

Any fish is allowed since most have approximately the same amount of protein. Although there are other protein sources that are not listed, such as bacon, other cheeses, and nuts, they are not considered good protein sources for a meal due to their high fat content. They may be used as an adjunct to a meal on occasion, but not as the sole protein source at a meal.

Protein supplements, such as powders or bars, may be used as alternative protein sources. Protein bars and powders can be used as a replacement for protein at a meal but not as an entire meal replacement. We could eat a large salad and a protein shake instead of chicken breast or tuna to increase the variety of foods consumed. These supplements offer the individual a quick and easy protein source that is pre-digested (broken down and therefore more easily absorbed), low in fat and carbohydrate. Many of the powders and bars are fortified with vitamins and minerals which increase their nutritional value. These supplements also taste great! There are flavors such as cookie dough and chocolate mint which can help satisfy a sweet craving without giving-in to foods that would disrupt the weight loss process and are generally filled with chemicals and additives.

When following the Naturopathic Diet, the protein content of the protein bar or powder should be at least double the carbohydrate, and the fat content should be no more than one quarter of the protein. Of particular importance here is to note that Canadian and American labeling of nutrients differs. If the bar or powder follows American labeling, the manufacturer does not need to include non-absorbable carbohydrates, such as gylcerine, in the total carbohydrate count. Although glycerine technically contains many carbohydrates, they pass right though the bowel without breaking down further and therefore do not increase blood sugar levels like other carbohydrates. In Canada, it is required to list glycerine and other such non-absorbable carbohydrates in the carbohydrate count. Some of the Canadian products will thus initially appear to have more carbohydrate than protein, but in actual fact, they are equal to the American labeled bars listing fewer carbohydrates.

Among bars meeting this requirement are Nitrotech (great flavors with no significant aftertaste), Solid Protein (a very dense bar so you only need a little to fill up), and Slim Down Bar (a lighter bar that has small crispy bits for a better texture). This bar contains an extract from a white kidney bean that inhibits the release of the enzymes that break down carbohydrates, so that the majority of the carbohydrates in this bar are not absorbed. Among powders are Proteins Plus (a great tasting whey protein powder that does not require a blender to mix and does not contain an artificial sweetener) and Slim Down Powder (a soy protein powder with few carbohydrates and fat, and a high amount of protein, which is difficult to find in a soy product, especially without a sweetener).

The following chart lists the approximate ratio of protein to fat in different protein sources. This chart allows us to make better food choices as we can determine the amount of fat contained in the diet.

Protein to Fat Ratios

Protein Source	Protein : Fat Ratio
Egg Whites	All protein, no fat!
Chicken Breast (skinless)	6 : 1
Turkey Breast (skinless)	11 : 1
Salmon (poached)	2 : 1
Tuna (in water)	24 : 1
Trout (grilled)	6 : 1
Beef Steak	2 : 1
Pork Loin	0.7 : 1
Soy	variable

Among the best sources of protein are the various soy foods, such as tofu, misso, and natto. Not only do these foods provide a ready, good source of protein for the Naturopathic Diet, they are usually 'organic' (without hormone additives or pesticide treatments) and their phytoestrogen content has been shown to be effective in preventing and treating hormone disorders, cancer, and high cholesterol. Soy foods are such a good source of protein that I've included a full chapter on them later in this book. Despite their value, soy foods vary greatly with respect to their ratio of protein to fat. Soy by nature is 60 – 70% fat. Due to this, many soy products are now made in low fat versions. For example, Yves soy burgers contain an 18:1 protein to fat ratio. However, regular extra firm tofu contains a 1:1.7 ratio of protein to fat. We need to read the labels and always choose the low fat version of soy products.

Carbohydrates and Glycemic Indices

We cannot just eat protein alone. Continual protein in high concentration by itself, without any carbohydrate, will stimulate ketosis, a starvation state in which the insulin and glucose levels are very low and glucagon levels rise. The liver produces a small amount of glucose and significant amounts of ketone bodies. All tissues can use ketones as fuel, and this helps prevent excess protein break down during prolonged starvation, but this state is unhealthy for the body, particularly the kidneys, so should be avoided. This is why we must add carbohydrates to the meal.

When considering carbohydrates, the 'glycemic index' of the food becomes very important. We know that all carbohydrates break down into sugar, so we must select those that produce it in lower amounts and at a slower rate. Now, a diet based strictly on very low glycemic index vegetables would be rather unpalatable, so this diet does allow a wider variety with increased flexibility even in stage one.

The glycemic index of food is a measure of the amount of sugar available in food to be delivered to the blood. The higher the glycemic index, the faster the sugar is transported into the blood. Different foods have different glycemic indices, and this is one of the keys to a weight loss or energy boosting program. Carbohydrates, especially simple carbohydrates, have a very high glycemic index. These foods will be broken down very quickly into sugar, which moves quickly into the blood, rapidly raising blood sugar levels. These foods include rice, potatoes, breads, and candy. There are foods, however, such as lettuce, mushrooms, and strawberries, which do contain carbohydrates but have much lower glycemic indices and will subsequently not raise blood sugar levels excessively.

There are certain carbohydrates that are permitted in unlimited quantities – salads and most vegetables. Certain vegetables contain too much starch or sugar and will increase your blood sugar levels, although some of these (carrots, for example) are permitted in stage one because they contain many beneficial nutrients. By cutting out all the restricted carbohydrates from our diet, we will have lowered our blood sugars sufficiently to enjoy some of these high-sugar vegetables, safely.

Good and Bad Carbohydrate Food Sources

The Naturopathic Diet does not restrict all carbohydrate consumption. Certain carbohydrates – most vegetables, for example – are, in fact, unrestricted. Although we may not want to eat 20 spears of asparagus at one sitting, we need not worry if we do, as it amounts to only 10 grams of carbohydrate. These foods contain our vitamins and minerals, and we need a lot of them. These foods also help prevent diseases such as colon cancer, so we do not want to limit them. These are the foods that fill up the rest of our plate and our stomach. Other carbohydrates are allowed with varying limits, depending largely on their glycemic indexes.

Unlimited Vegetables

Most vegetables, apart from the few listed below as restricted from the diet, are allowed in unlimited quantities and therefore can be consumed at will. In general vegetables are not restricted because

1. they contain very beneficial vitamins and minerals;
2. the carbohydrate content is relatively low;
3. the fiber content is relatively high.

This table shows the approximate carbohydrate content of different vegetables. It is clear we do not need to shy away from these vegetables as their carbohydrate content is relatively low – and their nutrient content is high. This chart is for information and reassurance, not to limit your intake!

Unlimited Vegetables

In both stage one and two, you can eat as much of these vegetables as you wish.

Vegetable	approx. 10 grams	approx. 30 grams
Asparagus	20 spears	60 spears
Broccoli (chopped)	8 cups	24 cups
Broccoli (frozen)	1 1/2 cups	5 cups
Cabbage	12 cups	unlimited
Carrots	2 large	6 large
Cauliflower	4 cups	10 cups
Cucumber	1 1/2 medium	4 medium
Eggplant	2 cups	6 cups
Lettuce	unlimited	unlimited
Mushrooms	4 cups	12 cups
Onion	3/4 cup	2 1/4 cups
Red Peppers	3/4 large	2 1/4 large
Spinach	unlimited	unlimited
Tomatoes	2 medium	6 medium
Yellow Peppers	2 cups	6 cups

Limited Vegetables and Legumes

The vegetables that are listed here are permitted but should only be consumed in smaller or less frequent quantities (once a week).

These vegetables are nutrient dense and contain a high amount of fiber, but they also contain a fair amount of sugar. This category of food also includes the legumes (beans and peas).

Limited Vegetables and Legumes

In stage one, it is best to limit these foods to one serving (10 grams), once per week.

Vegetables	approx. 10 grams (0.35 oz.)	approx. 30 grams (1 oz.)
Beets	3/4 cup	2 1/4 cup
Corn (canned)	1/4 cup	1/4 cup
Green peas	1/2 cup	1 1/2 cup
Split peas	1/4 cup	3/4 cup

Legumes	approx. 10 grams (0.35 oz.)	approx. 30 grams (1 oz.)
Black Beans	1/4 cup	3/4 cup
Chick Peas	1/4 cup	3/4 cup
Chili Beans	1/3 cup	1 cup
Kidney Beans	1/4 cup	3/4 cup
Lima Beans	1/3 cup	1 cup
Pimentos	1/4 cup	3/4 cup
Refried Beans	1/3 cup	1 cup
Wax Beans	1/4 cup	3/4 cup
White Beans	1/4 cup	3/4 cup

Restricted Vegetables

There are certain vegetables that are to be restricted in the Naturopathic Diet because they contain too much sugar. These vegetables are listed below with their corresponding carbohydrate content.

Restricted Vegetables

These vegetables are not allowed at all in stage one of the diet.

Vegetable	approx. 10 grams	approx. 30 grams
Parsnips	1/2 cup	1 1/2 cup
Pumpkin	3/4 cup	2 1/4 cups
Rutabaga	3/4 cup	2 1/4 cups
Squash	1 cup	3 cups
Sweet Potato (baked)	3/4 cup	2 1/4 cups
White Potato (baked)	1/6 cup	1/2 cup
French Fries	5 fries	15 fries
Yam (baked)	1/4 cup	3/4 cup

Fruits

Fruits, like vegetables, are carbohydrates. They are quite high in fructose, a sugar that is quickly converted into glucose and delivered to the blood. For this reason, the fruits are restricted to two per day during *stage one* of the diet. The fruit chosen should be a medium sized fruit. Any fruit except for the banana is allowed; the banana is restricted from the diet because it too high in starch and sugar. Berries and melons are allowed, with one 3/4 cup serving being the equivalent of one fruit. Berries and some of the melons are actually quite low in sugar and are therefore a great fruit choice.

Fruit juice counts as fruit! One glass of juice is the equivalent of one piece of fruit. When a juice is made, most of the fiber is removed, leaving what is essentially sugared water fortified with vitamins. It is better to eat your fruit rather than drinking it!

The following is a chart of several different fruits and their corresponding carbohydrate content. A medium sized fruit is considered for all fruits listed below. One cup of berries or cut fruit is the equivalent to one fruit.

Fruits

In stage one of the diet, any two fruits (except bananas) are allowed each day.

Apple	20 grams
Applesauce (unsweetened 1/2 cup)	15 grams
Apricots (3)	10 grams
Banana	30 grams
Blackberries (1 cup)	13 grams
Blueberries (1 cup)	15 grams
Cantaloupe (chopped 1 cup)	11.4 grams
Cherries (1 cup)	22 grams
Dates (2)	12 grams
Figs (1)	9.6 grams
Grapefruit	18 grams
Grapes (1 cup)	16 grams
Honeydew Melon (chopped 1 cup)	15.5 grams
Kiwi	8.7 grams
Mandarin Orange (1 cup)	24 grams
Mango (1 cup)	33 grams
Nectarine	14 grams
Orange	11.5 grams
Papaya	27 grams
Peach	8.5 grams
Pear	21 grams
Pineapple (1 cup)	17 grams

Plum	8.5 grams
Prunes (2)	10.5 grams
Raisins (1/2 cup)	56 grams
Raspberry (1 cup)	8.5 grams
Strawberry (1 cup)	6.5 grams
Tangerine	9.5 grams
Watermelon (1 cup)	11 grams

We need not concern ourselves with choosing only fruits that are very low in carbohydrate, but if we always gravitate towards those extremely high in carbohydrates, we will not lower our insulin secretion as quickly. For example, a half a cup of raisins contains 56 grams of carbohydrate, whereas an entire peach only contains 8.5 grams. This does not mean that we should never eat raisins, but we may not want to make them our daily fruit staple. The main restriction here is that we may not exceed two fruits a day.

Other Limited Carbohydrates

There are many foods that contain both protein and carbohydrate, such as yogurt, lentils, chickpeas, kidney beans, and other legumes. What is of particular importance here is the ratio of protein to carbohydrate. Throughout the diet, and particularly in stage one, a high concentration of protein is needed with a smaller amount of carbohydrate. Thus we want to choose foods that fit this balance. Yogurt has a carbohydrate to protein ratio of approximately 2:1, and kidney beans are 3:1. These foods are higher in carbohydrate than we would like. For this reason, these foods are to be considered carbohydrates and should therefore be limited.

Most cheeses (except cottage and ricotta, which are excellent protein sources), despite having an acceptable protein to carbohydrate ratio, are rather too high in fat to be consumed daily. A small amount of these food types are allowed, for instance a slice of cheese or a few chick peas on a salad, but do not eat them in excess or you will throw off your food group balance.

Similarly, if we eat these foods they must not be considered as a protein source. If we have some yogurt or lentils, we must still have another protein from the protein list at that meal. Our body will recognize these foods primarily as a carbohydrate and that is how we must treat them.

Forbidden Carbohydrates

Generally speaking, all foods with a high glycemic index should be eliminated from the diet in stage one. For quite obvious reasons, this category includes all grains and breads. These foods are purely carbohydrate, perhaps with a little fat, and will raise our blood sugar levels significantly. Many of these foods, such as rice or bread, seem quite harmless, but their breakdown into sugar is so quick that it is almost like ingesting pure sugar. For example, two thirds of a cup of white rice will produce the same reaction in your body as one half a cup of white sugar. It is for this reason that these foods must be completely eliminated during stage one of the Naturopathic Diet.

Therefore, no muffins, rolls, bagels, cereal, cookies, etc. If it is made from flour, it must be considered a grain or bread, even if that flour is ground from rice or spelt. These 'flour' foods must be avoided. The list of forbidden foods also includes potatoes, squash, yams, rice, pasta, popcorn, bananas, ice cream, and candy.

The following table illustrates the carbohydrate content of the restricted grains. It is easy to see why these carbohydrates are to be restricted in comparison with nutrient dense vegetables. If the two types of carbohydrates are compared on a 30 gram basis, eating 60 asparagus spears is much healthier than 3/4 cup of couscous, and 6 tomatoes are better than 1/2 waffle. Making more nutritious food choices not only leads to a healthier diet but also allows you to eat more!

Forbidden Carbohydrates

In stage one of the diet, these foods must be completely avoided.

Grain Carbohydrate	approx. 10 grams	approx. 30 grams
Bagel	1/3 bagel	1
Bread	1/2 piece	11/2 piece
Bun (hamburger or hotdog)	1/2 bun	11/2 buns
Couscous	1/4 cup	3/4 cup
Crackers (Saltine/Melba)	4 crackers	12 crackers
English Muffin	1/3 muffin	1 muffin
Oatmeal	1/4 cup	3/4 cup
Pancakes	1/2 cakes	1 1/2 cakes
Pasta	1/4 cup	3/4 cup
Pizza Crust (9 inch)	1/12 crust	1/4 crust
Rice (brown)	1/4 cup	3/4 cup
Rice (white)	1/4 cup	3/4 cup
Risotto	1/8 cup	1/4 cup
Tortilla	1 shell	3 shells
Waffle (7 inch)	1/4 waffle	1/2 waffle

Condiments (ketchup, mustard, mayonnaise, etc.)

Condiments are considered carbohydrates because they are basically made with flour or starch and water. Some condiments are higher in sugar, such as ketchup, while others, like curry paste, contain less. You may add any dressing, condiment, or spice that you wish to your food, but try to use these carbohydrate foods sparingly. The more sauce you put on your food, the higher the glycemic index of that food.

The Naturopathic Diet is meant to be enjoyed. We don't need to compromise taste for the sole purpose of restricting carbohydrate. If you restrict yourself too much, you will not enjoy the foods you are eating. But use your discretion when you spice up your foods!

Beverages

Alcoholic beverages are also a carbohydrate since most are made from fermented and distilled fruit or grains. For this reason, they, too, should be eliminated from the stage one of the Naturopathic Diet.

Most non alcoholic beverages are allowed on the protein diet. The consumption of any juice is permitted but it must be counted as one piece of fruit for that day. Soda pops or colas are allowed as well but they must be diet drinks. The amount of sugar in regular pop if far too great. Caffeinated drinks such as tea and coffee are also allowed. The addition of milk and sugar is admissible, but once again we must not overload our drink with unnecessary carbohydrates. If we are consuming several cups of coffee a day, the best solution is to try to cut down by switching to half caffeinated and half decaffeinated coffee so that we don't enter into caffeine withdrawal. Following this, we can slowly decrease the number of cups of coffee we drink without any side effects, while at the same time decreasing the amount of sugar we take in.

Caffeine and diet drinks, although permitted, are not the healthiest choice of fluids. Caffeine will further dehydrate our body in addition to the increased urination that occurs on a high protein diet. These lost fluids must be replaced. Water is the best beverage we can drink. It can be carbonated or flat, with some freshly squeezed lemon or lime added for flavor and to support the liver in the process of detoxification.

Stage One Summary:

✦ 15-25 grams of protein per meal.
✦ Unlimited salads and most vegetables.
✦ Maximum of 2 pieces of fruit a day. No bananas.
✦ No grains, rice, pastas or starches.
✦ Very limited high carbohydrate, low protein foods
(e.g. chickpeas, lentils)
✦ Watch portion used of dressings or condiments.
✦ No alcohol.
✦ Keep up fluid levels by drinking water.

Stage Two: The Weight Maintenance Stage

The maintenance stage of the naturopathic diet is a true lifestyle pattern that we can easily maintain for the rest of our life. Throughout this second stage, our energy levels will remain high, our weight stable. We can enjoy every food group and continue to protect ourselves against many food related diseases at the same time. These benefits will last forever as long as we balance our protein and newly introduced carbohydrates at each meal. The maintenance stage is thus not so much a stage as it is a permanent change.

During stage two we begin to reintroduce some of the carbohydrates that were eliminated or markedly reduced in stage one. Now that our body has consolidated the protein/low glucose message, it is possible to add in carbohydrates at a higher concentration, along with the protein, without increasing insulin release. Blood sugar levels will not rise rapidly as they did before, the reason being that the protein we are combining with the carbohydrates will slow the delivery of the sugar into the blood. This in itself will reduce the amount of insulin released. In addition, the reversal of insulin resistance and hyperinsulinemia achieved by stage one will further reduce the insulin response. Overall less insulin will be secreted than before we started the diet. This will inhibit weight gain. Slightly more insulin will be released during stage two than during stage one, and this will prevent further weight loss.

When we reintroduce the carbohydrates we will stop losing weight. We will not regain the weight we have lost, but the stage one weight loss process will stop. We may never ingest carbohydrates at the rate we did before or we may wish to incorporate them at every meal. The choice is ours.

The order in which we reintroduce the carbohydrates is very important. We must slowly integrate them back into the diet in a particular pattern. The sequence of reintroduction is determined by the glycemic index and type of sugar found in each carbohydrate. Fructose, the sugar found in fruit, is the first to be introduced. Then glucose from whole grains and breads, followed by pasta, rice, then potatoes and squash, and finally candy and alcohol. Following this approach minimizes large jumps in blood sugar levels and allows for easy adaptation of the body to carbohydrates.

Reintroduction Order

1. Fruits
2. Whole Grains, Breads, Cereals
3. Pasta
4. Rice
5. Potatoes and Squash
6. Candy and Alcoholic Beverages

The amount of carbohydrate that you bring back into the diet is also very important. We must maintain a balance between carbohydrates and protein at each meal in order to preserve the biochemical changes we have brought about during stage one. While a specific amount of carbohydrate cannot be quoted because it differs from individual to individual, as a general rule, a ratio of one part protein to one part carbohydrate, excluding vegetables and salads, is a fairly good balance.

We should reintroduce a small amount of carbohydrate initially, approximately three parts protein to one part carbohydrate at each meal (for example, 21 grams protein with 7 grams carbohydrate). We should remain at this level of carbohydrate intake for four to five days. A typical meal would be half a slice of bread, a piece of chicken, and unlimited salad or vegetable.

During this time period, we need to watch for signs of hyperinsulinemia. Our body will become symptomatic when we ingest too many carbohydrates at once. We will feel tired shortly after the meal as our blood sugar levels drop too low. Several hours later or perhaps the next day we may feel bloated as our kidneys are not releasing enough salt. These signs will let us know that the ratio of carbohydrate to protein was too high and therefore insulin was secreted at a higher rate.

If none of these signs appear following the amount of reintroduced carbohydrate, then we can increase the amount consumed
again. This time we might consider a ratio of 2:1 protein to carbohydrate. Again we need to watch for signs and symptoms of hyperinsulinemia. If they do not appear, we a can continue to increase slowly
the amount and type of carbohydrate until we have reached a 1:1
ratio. Should the symptoms of hyperinsulinemia appear earlier, we
have discovered our limit of carbohydrate intake and must return to
the proportion previously used where no symptoms occurred.

This is our state of dietary balance. This is the ratio of protein to
carbohydrate that we can ingest without changing our weight ever.
At this balance between protein and carbohydrate, our blood sugar
levels will remain steady and subsequently so will our insulin secretion and weight.

Stage Two Summary:

➤ Continue 15-25 grams protein per meal.
➤ Continue unlimited salad/vegetable.
➤ Carbohydrate reintroduction:
1. Type - follow reintroduction order listed above
2. Amount - slowly reintroduce carbohydrates starting at a
ratio of 3 protein : 1 carbohydrate
3. Increase - slowly increase the proportion of carbohydrate
to protein towards 1:1
4. Watch for symptoms of hyperinsulinemia - If symptoms appear
return to previous ratio at which no symptoms occurred
THIS is your own personal protein solution!

Rate of Weight Loss

The rate of weight loss, as with any change in the body, will vary among people, but on average there is a two pound weight loss per week. During the first week, this may double or triple, with half of that loss being attributed to water. It is quite common to see larger losses one week followed by a smaller loss in the second. Some individuals even see large losses of 4 to 5 pounds a week for 2 to 3 weeks. This is usually followed by a plateau period or a decrease in the rate of loss back to around two pounds per week.

This is very safe and manageable level of weight loss. If it were any faster, it would begin to drain our body of energy and place stress on other areas such as the immune system and the adrenal glands (stress glands). If it were any slower, it would be frustrating.

Most individuals continue losing weight at this rate until they are ready to move into the maintenance phase. However, there are a few people who may plateau during the diet. If it is a one week plateau, then it is of no significance. If it is three or more weeks, then we may want to consider augmenting the diet with natural supplements such as herbs, vitamins, or minerals to safely speed up the weight loss, but always remember, if you lose weight too quickly, your body will get tired and not function quite as well. Supplements are not needed if we are maintaining a two pound per week loss. These supplements are discussed later in the book.

Health Benefits and Positive Side Effects

When followed correctly, there are usually only positive side effects with the Naturopathic Diet. Many of these effects we may not notice, such as an improvement in our immune system function or faster and stronger growing nails and hair. There are some changes that virtually everyone on the diet experiences and these are due to physiological changes that result from high protein. Other not so common changes seen are usually due to differences in lifestyles and or previous diets. Just as we don't all react to medications in the same way, we don't all react to dietary changes in the same manner.

Weight Loss

The first significant health benefit of the Naturopathic Diet is weight loss. Everyone who follows stage one of the diet will notice this within the first week. Once again, the amount of weight loss will vary slightly among individuals, but the average loss is two pounds a week with a larger loss in the first week. Even if you are not trying to lose weight, this diet can be used for its beneficial effects on energy level and the cardiovascular system. The diet will help slim patients to better control the use of their food. However, as there tends to be a substantial initial weight loss, stage one is limited in these individuals to 7 to 10 days. Once glucose and insulin levels are stabilized, the individual moves rapidly to stage two, the maintenance stage, thereby avoiding further weight loss.

Increased Energy Level

An increase in energy level is felt by almost everyone on the diet due to the establishment of consistent blood sugar levels. It is very energetically taxing on the body to have blood sugar levels rise high and then fall precipitously, forcing our metabolism to work inefficiently and harder with fewer beneficial results. When our sugar levels remain constant, we no longer get those dips in energy, and an even delivery of sugar to the blood between meals is assured, thus keeping energy levels just as constant.

Some individuals do experience a decrease in energy during the first week due to the adjustment in their diet, but this side effect soon passes. The body is now receiving an entirely new type of food, a useable food, but a new food nonetheless. No longer is there a sugar rush after each meal, and it was this rush that resulted in a 'high' feeling. After the sugar crash, the body demanded another sugar fix, resulting in another high. People on the Naturopathic Diet no longer experience highs and lows, but if we are used to the highs, an absence of them may feel bad. This feeling is short-lived as the body adapts to its new metabolism and energy levels remain constant.

Improved Digestion

Changes in the digestive system are always seen. A new food type is being used, one that is more easily digested, making breakdown more efficient in the bowel. If you take a look at different bowel disorders, there are no diseases due to improper breakdown of vegetables or protein, but there are a number of disorders related to the way the bowel deals with grains. For instance, in celiac disease individuals cannot digest the gluten in grains, and Crohn's disease has been shown to result in poor breakdown of dissaccharides (sugars) in simple carbohydrates. There are numerous other bowel conditions in which grains and starches adversely affect the digestive tract.

On the Naturopathic Diet there is a dramatic decrease in gas and bloating. Reversal of the hyperinsulinemia allows the kidneys to release salt and water. Foods eaten are more easily digested and therefore very little undigested food passes through the bowel. It is undigested food that the bacteria in the gut feed upon, resulting in gas and bloating. As well, we are no longer ingesting the bulking foods like breads and pastas.

The vegetables and fruit that are readily consumed on the protein diet are very high in fiber. Despite the fact that individuals on the diet are no longer eating the high-fiber grains, they will be ingesting enough, if not more fiber, than they did before, so bowel movements will remain easy and soft. If bowel movements were firm before, they should become more loose and easier to pass. This is due not only to the high fiber and fluid loss through the bowel, but also due to the nature of the fiber type itself. No longer are you consuming large amounts of bulking fiber, so the stool will not be as voluminous. In some people this may lead to less frequent bowel emptying as the intestines no longer need to rid themselves of all this bulk. There should be no problem with constipation on this diet. If there is any feeling of constipation, it is usually because fluids levels are not being maintained. Simply increasing the amount of water intake should rectify the situation very quickly.

Lowered Insulin Levels

An increase in urination is usually seen in most people following the protein diet. The decrease in insulin allows the kidneys to release excess salt the body was holding. Water always follows salt, and therefore you will release the extra fluids through urination. Some people experience an increase in flow at each urination, others have an increased frequency. Either way, this is a good sign for we know that insulin levels are being lowered when this is seen.

Detoxification

When we begin the Naturopathic Diet, our body will begin to detoxify quite slowly because we are no longer eating 'toxic' foods like candy and muffins that are loaded with all sorts of additives and preservatives which the liver must process. When the toxic load is lightened on the liver, it will begin to clear itself and the blood of any toxins that may be lingering from our previous dietary habits. Similarly, toxins outside the liver are stored in our fat. As the fat breaks down and we lose weight, these toxins are released into the blood stream and cleared by the liver. For these reasons a good water intake is essential. Water helps to flush out those toxins and cleans the body as we proceed on the Naturopathic Diet.

Prevention and Treatment of Disease

The most important side effect of all is one that we will not see – the prevention (or treatment if we had a prior food related disease) of diabetes, hypertension, high cholesterol, and heart disease. This is the most powerful side effect of all and at the same time the one we are usually least concerned about as it does not have an impact on us today. Just as the weight that we lose is a permanent change, so is the improvement in health.

The Naturopathic Diet has proven to be therapeutic in my medical practice. On several occasions patients have come to me taking several different medications for high blood pressure, high cholesterol, and blood sugar control. They have been told to change their diet and lose weight but have usually not been given any direction. Most people begin on their own by cutting out the fat and therefore most protein sources with it. Once again they default to a high carbohydrate diet. Even those individuals who stick mostly to fruits and vegetables as their carbohydrates still continue to gain weight and are certainly no closer to improving their health. Only once they understand the impact that protein has on their health and their pre-existing conditions do they start to see positive effects.

Tony Bell, a 55-year-old man, presented with high cholesterol and was advised to take drugs to help lower this. With reluctance, his family doctor agreed to hold off, provided that Tony change his diet, lose weight, and continue monitoring his cholesterol. After two months on the Naturopathic Diet, Tony's 'bad' cholesterol had dropped 3 points, back down to the low end of the normal range, and his 'good' cholesterol, HDL, had risen 1 point. After seeing this result, Tony's family doctor and I now have a wonderful relationship. He advises most of his patients to go on the Naturopathic Diet first before trying pharmaceutical medications.

A similar case was that of Mary Walborough, who was experiencing chest tightness, high blood pressure, and fatigue. After a thorough work up from her family doctor, she was diagnosed with beginning stages of arteriosclerosis, high blood pressure, and obesity. After 4 months of the Naturopathic Diet, not only did Mary lose 45 pounds, but she had no more chest pain, and her blood pressure dropped from 152/96 to 118/77. Once again Mary was able to regain control of her health and help to prevent further damage to her heart, arteries, and the rest of her body.

Safety

The Naturopathic Diet can be used safely by almost everyone, regardless of age or state of health. It is wonderful for children because there are some great tasting high protein recipes they will love. Most children do not eat enough protein. It took years to create our weight problem, and it all began when we were young. The Naturopathic Diet will help prevent our children from facing the same weight gain problem we are now battling.

Similarly, the elderly can profit greatly from this diet. Protein is a major constructive substrate in our immune system, strengthening our immune function, which is of particular importance in the elderly.

Studies have shown that high performance athletes benefit greatly from a diet such as this. Their bodies learn to tap into their fat as a fuel source and use their food more efficiently. An elite athlete who is training several hours a day may want to increase the protein and carbohydrate intake considerably. The best way for an athlete to introduce this diet into a training regime is to initiate it at the beginning of the season or even before the season starts. Again, stage one is short so they will already be in the maintenance phase, which is higher in carbohydrate, before they start racing. Performance will improve as metabolic output is optimized.

There are a few cases and disease conditions, however, in which the protein diet needs to modified slightly and monitored by a health care practitioner.

1. Renal Disease: Any individual with renal (kidney) disease or who only has one kidney must be careful on a high protein diet. Protein is quite high in phosphorus, and if you overload a damaged kidney with too much phosphorus, it is possible to cause further damage. That does not mean that people with renal damage or one kidney cannot use the protein diet; it simply

means that they must use smaller protein ratios and must consult with a health practitioner before doing so.

2. Diabetes: This diet program is perfect for the diabetic individual as it keeps blood sugar levels at the low end of normal, but diabetics on insulin will have to adjust insulin intake as they proceed with this diet. Most likely insulin intake will have been adjusted to a diet that is high in carbohydrates, assuming that blood sugar levels are equally as high. Therefore, close monitoring of blood sugar levels and insulin dose is required. Diabetics might want to seek a little help from a health care practitioner in this regard.

3. Weight Disorders: For people who are very underweight, medical monitoring is recommended, though I have seen great results with this diet even in anorexic and bulimic patients as they can eat a healthy diet without feeling "heavy" or bloated. In these cases, however, I consider counseling or psychological support essential to deal with underlying issues.

The only negative side effect from the Naturopathic Diet is the feeling of a 'foggy head' sensation a few individuals experience. When there is an increased urine output, certain electrolytes are lost in greater amounts. One, in particular, is potassium. This is a very important electrolyte as it is used to maintain proper electrolyte balance in the blood and to control proper functioning of the heart and brain. If the potassium lost in the urine is not replaced, a foggy or groggy head feeling may result. Because any high protein product will increase urination, most protein powders or bars supplement with extra potassium to eliminate this feeling. If proper potassium levels are maintained, which is very easy to do, then no side effect is seen.

This is one of the reasons why the Naturopathic Diet includes nutritional supplements to assist in safe weight loss and healthy weight maintenance.

Nutritional Supplementation

How Much Supplementation?

Vitamins, Minerals & Herbs

Required Weight Loss Supplements

Potassium

Calcium

Magnesium

Vitamin B-1

Vitamin B-2

Vitamin B-3

Vitamin B-6

Vitamin B-12

Vitamin B 'Complex'

Weight Loss Enhancing Supplements

Phosphates

Guggul Lipids

L-Carnitine

Garcinia Cambogia

Citrus Aurantium

Conjugated Linoleic Acid (CLA)

Biotin

Pausinystalia Yohimba

Chromium

NUTRITIONAL SUPPLEMENTATION

Nutritional supplementation is the addition of vitamins and minerals to the diet for preventative and therapeutic purposes. This philosophy of supplementation has been gradually gaining more acceptance over the past few years as we are becoming more aware of the deficiencies in our food. Not only are our 'fast-food' food choices lacking in vitamins and minerals, even our supposedly fresh vegetables and fruit are nutrient depleted. Our farm soils are exhausted, no longer enriched with natural minerals. Supposedly fresh foods have usually spent many days in storage or transport before making it to our plates. Food storage and processing generally destroys over 50% of the vitamin/mineral content in that food, though variations exist between different nutrients within the food. Baking obliterates 100% of vitamin B-1, while processing damages 80% of vitamin B-2. Given our over-processed, stale, nutrient-scarce diets it is easy to see why nutrient supplementation has grown in popularity.

How Much Supplementation?

G uidelines have been developed by the U.S.A. Food and Drug Administration and other national health organizations to generalize the amount of nutrients necessary for all the different bodily functions. This measurement is known as the RDA, the Recommended Dietary Allowance. These values are designed to simplify supplementation and give a daily average amount of required nutrients for the general population. The problem with this is that we are all different. The concentration of vitamins and minerals required by each individual is slightly different as we all place different demands upon our bodies and have different underlying genetic make-ups. Similarly, lifestyle plays a major role in the amount of nutrient we each require. A smoker will need twice as much vitamin C and a very stressed individual will require extra vitamin B complex. As a result, we all must supplement somewhat differently.

Regardless of these individual differences, the recommended amount of supplementation per day is generally far too low. Recent nutritional research has discovered that the optimal level for many nutrients is much higher than that suggested by the RDA values. Some of this need may have been brought about by a changing environment, such as the depleted soils forming nutrient-scarce food or the rise in pollution necessitating extra protection. While following the RDA values for nutrient supplementation we will most likely prevent the majority of nutrition-deficient diseases, such as pellegra (vitamin B-3 deficiency) or scurvy (inadequate vitamin C), we will not be allowing our bodies to function at maximum levels and will therefore never reach optimal health.

Vitamins, Minerals & Herbs

Vitamins are defined as any constituents in the diet other than protein, fat, carbohydrate, and inorganic salts that are necessary for normal growth and activity of the body. They must be obtained from external sources, and a deficiency may result in specific diseases depending on the vitamin.

Minerals are essentially any inorganic substance found in the earth. Like vitamins, minerals must be taken in from an outside source and are necessary for proper bodily maintenance and growth. Minerals can be divided into two categories. *Macrominerals* are those that the body needs in larger doses of milligrams or even grams. This includes such minerals as calcium, magnesium, phosphorus, and potassium. *Trace minerals* are those which are required in much smaller amounts, in micrograms. This category includes iodine, selenium, and chromium, for example.

Herbs, simply put, are plants or plant products, typically the flower, leaf, or root of a plant. The medicinal properties of herbs have been recognized for many centuries, and were used extensively by the ancient Egyptians. Pharmaceutical medicine developed from the use of these herbs, as the different plant products were then isolated and made available in a purer and more potent form. Herbs contain healing properties just as drugs do and it is very important to control their use and dose. However, when used correctly, herbal medicine becomes a very powerful tool at enhancing the body's functions, repairing injury, and regulating disease.

Vitamins and minerals are essential components of enzymes and coenzymes. Enzymes are substances that stimulate different biochemical reactions in the body. Coenzymes aid the enzymes in this function. With proper nutritional supplementation, we can support certain enzymatic pathways to perform optimally, thereby speeding up certain reactions. If an enzyme is lacking a vitamin or mineral, it cannot function optimally and the process is slowed or halted. We must therefore ensure adequate nutrient supplementation to accentuate certain bodily functions.

This idea may be applied to weight loss. Through specific supplementation, we can enhance the metabolic reactions in the body and maximize weight loss. Supplements are not to be considered an alternative to the diet. Supplements will not teach your body's metabolism the vital lessons of proper food breakdown and energy use. They simply aid in the weight loss process. If we use only the supplements and do not follow the Naturopathic Diet, our body will not learn how to metabolize our food for energy instead of storing it as fat. Upon cessation of the supplements, we will most likely gain back all of the weight we lost, if not more.

Required Weight Loss Supplements

Certain vitamins and minerals are necessary during the diet, for metabolic and electrolyte balance. They also aid in the processing of food.

Potassium

Potassium is a mineral that is required throughout the duration of the Naturopathic Diet. It is a positively charged electrolyte that is very important for proper brain, muscle, nerve, kidney, and heart functioning. This mineral is lost in high rates in the urine during the weight loss portion of the Naturopathic Diet and thus should be supplemented. Due to the fact that urination is increased greatly from the drop in insulin, more potassium than normal is lost and must be replaced. Many high protein products such as protein drinks or bars are supplemented with potassium for this reason. If you are using these products daily, you may not need to add extra potassium in pill form. If you are not receiving enough potassium from your food, you may experience that 'foggy head' feeling discussed earlier.

Potassium may be taken at any time of the day, with food. Most potassium supplements are sold in 99 mg tablets. There is no problem taking all 99 mg, even if we only need 50 mg. Our body will rid itself of a little extra potassium in the urine or in our sweat. If we are experiencing a foggy head feeling and we are already taking 100 mg, we can safely increase this amount. This supplement is best taken with food to minimize stomach upset.

Recommended dose: 50-100 mg/day

Calcium

Calcium is an essential mineral. It helps to regulate blood pressure, prevent osteoporosis, reduce muscle cramps, and much more. Due to the fact that calcium is used all over the body, if our blood or tissue calcium levels drop, our body will catabolize (break down) our bone to replenish it and to maintain proper bodily functioning. When following a high protein diet, more muscle is usually formed and therefore more calcium is usually required to sustain muscle growth, repair, and function.

As well, calcium and phosphorus compete with each other in different bodily processes. A diet high in phosphorus may deplete calcium stores. Protein is high in phosphorus, so we must once again ensure extra calcium intake to counteract the loss through the elevated dietary phosphorus. This becomes particularly important for those women who are trying to maintain maximum bone quantity and quality.

Recommended dose: for women 1000-1200mg/day

for men 500-750 mg/day

Magnesium

Magnesium is essential to the functioning of over 300 enzymes in the body. These enzymes are used for breaking down glucose, muscle contraction, energy production, and many other functions. Magnesium is a mineral that functions closely with calcium. The two work together to control muscle activity and prevent spasms. Recent studies show that many muscle disorders, such as fibromyalgia or chronic muscle pain, are associated with magnesium deficiency. As well, low blood levels of magnesium have been consistently seen in fatigue. Due to the importance of proper muscle function in fat metabolism, it is easy to see the benefits of magnesium supplementation throughout life but especially during a high protein diet.

Calcium and magnesium can be taken together in one supplement. Most formulas will require you to take two or three pills a day to obtain the recommended dose. These minerals can be taken with or without food, and at least one dose should be taken before bed. While you sleep certain hormones are secreted that will maximize calcium absorption.

Recommended dose: 500 to 750 mg/day

Vitamin B-1

Vitamin B-1 or thiamin is a water soluble vitamin. It is a constituent of an enzyme called thiamin pyrophosphate and is required for oxidative decarboxylation of alpha keto-acids. What this actually means is that vitamin B-1 helps to breakdown carbohydrates, thus creating energy. It also has a specific role aiding nerve cell function. Due to its role in carbohydrate metabolism, vitamin B-1 is a recommended supplement for a high-protein diet.

Recommended dose: 50 to 100 mg/day

Vitamin B-2

Vitamin B-2, also known as riboflavin, is also a water soluble vitamin. Riboflavin is necessary for the production of energy and burning of fat as it helps to increase mitochondrial output. Once again the mitochondria are the components in muscle that are responsible for breaking down fat and generating both heat and energy. Vitamin B-2 is thus another vitamin important for weight loss.

Apart from the metabolic benefits of vitamin B-2, it is also involved in recycling glutathione, the main free radical quencher in the body that protects us from damaging pollutants. Low levels of riboflavin have been connected with certain cancers, especially esophageal cancer.

Recommended dose: 50 to 100 mg/day

Vitamin B-3

Vitamin B-3 (niacin or niacinamide) is used in the maintenance of blood sugar levels, the process of detoxification, the production of energy, and the reduction of cholesterol levels. It functions as part of two enzymes, NAD (nicotinamide adenine dinucleotide) and NADP (nicotinaminde adenine dinucleotide phosphate). These enzymes are part of the glycogen cycle where fatty acids are oxidized into energy.

Recommended dose: 30 to 80 mg/day

Vitamin B-6

Vitamin B-6 or pyridoxine, like the other B vitamins, is water soluble. This vitamin has been extensively studied and is now considered one of the most important vitamins available. It is utilized in many different bodily processes, including the production of hemoglobin and all new protein. As well, it helps to regulate nerve conduction, combat depression (as it is necessary for the manufacturing of serotonin, our body's 'happy' hormone), and prevent osteoporosis through the regulation of collagen cross-linking within the bone matrix. As it pertains to a high protein diet, vitamin B-6 is needed to help monitor the breakdown of protein and the synthesis of new proteins.

Recommended dose: 50-100 mg/day

Vitamin B-12

Vitamin B-12, also known as cyanocobalamin, functions more with coenzymes than it does with enzymes. It is essential for the growth of all new cells and is used in energy metabolism and immune function while aiding in proper nerve transmission throughout the body. Due to its role in cell growth and energy metabolism, vitamin B-12 is a very useful vitamin to supplement with during this diet.

Recommended dose: 50-100 mcg/day

Vitamin B 'Complex'

A combination of B vitamins can be taken in a multi B supplement. This supplement should contain a minimum of 50 mg (milligrams) of each B, except B-12, which should be 50 mcg (micrograms). The supplement will most likely include all the B's mentioned above as well as B-5 or pantothenic acid.

One to two of these should be taken a day *with food* ; a vitamin B supplement may irritate a stomach if it is empty. When taking a vitamin B-1 or vitamin B complex supplement, your urine may turn a fluorescent yellow color. Do not panic! Vitamin B-1 has a yellow-green pigment that, when mixed with water, will color the water yellow.

Weight Loss Enhancing Supplements

The human body always strives to stay in a homeostatic balance; it does not always like change even if it is good for us. As our body changes throughout a diet, it may start to fight this change. This is known as the 'diet plateau' where the weight loss temporarily halts. This plateau usually lasts a couple of weeks and then the weight loss commences once again. However, in certain individuals it is more difficult to break that plateau as the body continues to fight change. It may be necessary in these people to re-stimulate the weight loss process through herbal or other nutritional supplementation. For those who continue to lose weight, it is not necessary to use these supplements. These supplements are for those individuals in whom the protein diet alone does not result in the expected weight loss. Just as hair color or leg length vary between people, so does their response to a diet. It is nice to know that there is a solution for those people who need a little extra help.

Phosphates

As blood sugar levels stabilize on the naturopathic diet, most people feel less hungry and therefore eat less. The food that we eat is used to manufacture ATP, the body's energy substrate. When there are fewer calories taken into the body, less ATP is formed. If ATP production drops below a certain level, this level differing among people, it may result in a decrease in thyroid output. Our thyroid is the gland responsible for controlling our metabolic rate. By lowering its output, we can lower the rate at which we burn fat. This is why calorie-depriving, crash diets alter metabolism and slow or halt weight loss.

The key to *healthy* weight loss is to maintain normal ATP production so that the thyroid will also continue to function at its optimal rate. This can be achieved in one of two ways. First, we can eat more food; however, assuming that we are already taking in the required protein and good carbohydrates, we will be receiving more than enough nutrients to maintain a healthy body. Taking in more food will only add extra calories. The other solution is to increase the body's production of ATP by providing it with more of the constituents that make up ATP, phosphates.

Phosphates are minerals that we get through regular diet. By supplementing with extra phosphates, we can help to maintain normal ATP levels in the liver and send the appropriate message to the thyroid. Phosphate supplementation will not increase thyroid hormone levels unless the thyroid output is already reduced. It will only return thyroid function back to normal and not abnormally increase your metabolic rate. Too many phosphates may damage your kidneys, however.

Phosphate supplements are to be used only by people who are eating only the basic protein requirement and can therefore handle the extra supplementation. If the protein intake is on the high end of the allowed range mentioned in the protein section, phosphate supplementation is not recommended. For these individuals, extra phosphates are not usually required as protein itself is high in phosphorus.

Phosphate supplementation is contraindicated in any individual with poor kidney function.

Recommended dose: 500 mg twice a day with food

Guggul Lipids

Guggul lipids were first introduced as a means of reducing cholesterol in the liver. They have since been shown to stimulate thyroid hormone output, once again maximizing this gland's potential to control our metabolism. Guggul lipids contain active ingredients known as guggulsterones that can increase T3 and T4 output. T3 and T4 are our thyroid hormones that are produced by the thyroid gland. They are ultimately responsible for the actions of that gland, playing a major role in the control of our metabolism and ultimately weight loss. With guggul lipid supplementation, clinical studies reveal normalization of metabolic rate in those whose thyroid output was deficient.

Recommended dose: 500 mg, three times a day on an
empty stomach

L-Carnitine

Carnitine is a trimethylated carboxyl alcohol which exists in three forms. L-carnitine bound to acetic acid (LAC) mimics the neurotransmitter acetylcholine and is therefore used mostly with the elderly or in brain disorders. L-carnitine bound to proprionic acid (LPC) is the form that the heart prefers and is therefore used in different cardiovascular diseases. Unbound L-carnitine is used most freely by the body. L-carnitine helps to transport long fatty acid chains throughout the body. Fat is not burned at the same place it is stored. Fat is broken down in the mitochondria of muscle cells. However, fat cannot just move over to those mitochondria by itself – it needs a carrier. L-carnitine acts as its transport mechanism delivering the fat to the muscle so that it may be used as energy.

Although our bodies normally manufacture L-carnitine in the liver, kidneys, and brain, it is not always in sufficient concentration. The higher the concentration of L-carnitine in the muscle, the more fat that can be burned. Once again supplementation of a specific nutrient can aid a specific pathway an optimize weight loss.

As with other supplements, we do not want to over stimulate one pathway. The body functions as a whole unit so that a change in one area may create a change in another. L-carnitine supplementation, like the other nutrients, should only be used to optimize body processes, not to elevate them above their normal function.

Recommended dose: 800-1500 mg/day

Garcinia Cambogia

Garcinia cambogia is a fruit grown in southern India which contains a compound known as hydroxycitric acid (HCA). This acid has been clinically proven to reduce weight through two different mechanisms. *Garcinia cambogia* is used to inhibit a process known as lipogenesis. Lipogenesis is the formation of fat from the different foods that we eat. It also includes the deposition of this fat into the adipose tissue of the body. Despite the fact that HCA can prevent the formation of excess fat from food, it does so without altering protein metabolism. Once again, lean body tissue is preserved for maximum fat burning potential.

The second role that *garcinia cambogia* plays in weight loss is as an appetite suppressant. HCA stimulates a feeling of satiety and satisfaction earlier in a meal, thereby reducing the amount of food eaten at one time. Not only does this lower the calorie intake, but it lessens the demand placed on the digestive tract. When too much food is consumed at once, not all of it is broken down, so undigested food passes into the bowel where it is fed upon by the bacterial flora. This in turn causes gas, bloating, and malabsorption.

Recommended dose: 350-500 mg directly after a meal

Citrus Aurantium

Citrus aurantium, better known as bitter orange, has a thermogenic effect that enables the body to mobilize fat more effectively so that it can be carried to the mitochondria (fat burners). It has also been shown to maximize the metabolic rate, thereby increasing the rate at which calories are burned.

This herb will only support and stimulate the metabolic rate up to its optimum function. It will not increase metabolism above normal levels.

Recommended dose: 150 mg, 30 minutes before a meal

Conjugated Linoleic Acid (CLA)

Conjugated Linoleic Acid or CLA is a previously unrecognized nutrient with wide variety of functions that occurs naturally in a wide variety of foods. Linoleic acid is an essential fatty acid known as an omega 6 fatty acid. It is used primarily to reduce pain and inflammation, and to regulate hormone production, blood pressure, and heart function. As well, CLA has anticarcinogenic and antioxidant properties.

In the context of weight loss, it is primarily used for its anticatabolic effect and as a growth hormone regulator. CLA prevents the loss of muscle tissue as is protects against a suppressed immune response during intense exercise or weight loss. Studies reveal that subjects supplemented with essential fatty acids and placed on an intense exercise and diet regime maintained their lean body tissue mass and were far less tired than those who were not given the supplementation. This suggests that essential fatty acid supplementation, primarily linoleic acid, helps to offset some of the negative effects of exercise and weight loss, such as decreased strength and immune function.

Recommended dose: 2000 mg/day

Biotin

Biotin is considered a B vitamin that functions in the manufacturing and utilization of fats and amino acids. It is available as an isolated form or a biocytin, a complex from brewers' yeast that contains 65.6% biotin. Biotin's main role in the body is to function as an essential enzymatic cofactor. It works primarily with four different enzymes, all of which add a carboxyl group to another molecule. This process, known as carboxylation, is vital in the metabolism of sugar, fats, and amino acids.

Biotin has long been used in the treatment of diabetes as it enhances insulin function and increases the activity of glucokinase. Glucokinase is an enzyme used in the breakdown of glucose by the liver for energy. Supplementation of biotin has been shown to lower significantly fasting blood sugar levels and improve the use of blood glucose. Biotin enables the body to use the sugar in the blood for fuel rather than storing it as fat.

Recommended dose: 200-250 mcg/day

Pausinystalia Yohimba (Yohimbe)

Pausinystalia yohimba, also known as yohimbe, is a tree indiginous to West Africa, specifically the Congo and Cameroon. The bark of this tree contains a mixture of different alkoloids; the principal alkoloid is yohimbine. Yohimbine has been used for many decades as a herb to help impotence. In 1990 it received FDA (Food and Drug Administration) approval, and since then has been widely distributed by herbal and pharmaceutical companies.

Yohimbine functions through two different mechanisms. First, it increases dilation of blood vessels in the skin and mucous membranes, thereby lowering blood pressure and decreasing impotence in men where it relates to lowered vascular flow. Second, yohimbine belongs to a class of substances known as alpha-2-receptor antagonists. These compounds cause a large increase in noradrenalin output from nerve endings. This in turn raises the body's core temperature and causes the mobilization of fat or fuel. It therefore is used as a thermogenic (heat producing) herb which induces the breakdown and utilization of fat. Not all thermogenic herbs cause the degradation of fat. Some herbs, like ginger or curcumin which have been added to weight loss formulas, simply increase circulation and therefore generate heat. These later herbs are very beneficial for the clearance of mucous during colds, for example, but have not yet been studied as they pertain to weight loss.

Recommended dose: 1-5 mg/day

Chromium

Chromium is a mineral that was first nicknamed the 'glucose tolerance factor'. It is now known that chromium is not a glucose factor itself, but rather an active factor in blood sugar control mechanisms. Chromium functions quite intimately with insulin in the uptake of glucose from the blood. Chromium's main role is to help insulin function properly so that it only takes the appropriate amount of glucose from the blood at any given time. As well, chromium plays a role in stimulating thermogenesis, the physiological production of heat in the body.

Clinically, chromium deficiency has been implicated in insulin irregularities, hypercholesterolemia, and high triglyceride levels. Similarly, chromium supplementation has been shown to lower body fat and preserve lean body tissue effectively.

There are several forms of chromium, including chromium polynicotinate, chromium chloride, chromium picolinate, and chromium-enriched yeasts. Most studies have been performed using chromium picolinate and therefore this form is most widely used.

Recommended dose: 200 mcg/day

Herbal Combination Supplements

Several natural supplement companies have prepared herbal supplements designed to assist with weight loss. One supplement combination that has been very effective with many of my patients is Ultra Slim Down by Jamieson Vitamins, which combines several natural supplements. It is comprised of two separate products. The first is a combination of HCA, Avantra-Ztm, and Kola nut, to be taken 30 minutes before a meal to help prepare the body biochemically for the food to be ingested. HCA or hydroxycitric acid, derived from the fruit of the Garcinia Cambogia tree, is an herbal carbohydrate burner that assists the body in converting dietary carbohydrates into energy rather than into fat. Advantra-Ztm, derived from bitter orange, helps mobilize fat more efficiently, making it easier to burn. A decaffeinated version of Kola nut is used to help increase energy levels by supporting the adrenal or stress glands. The second product is a combination of two fiber sources, Chitosan and Napal cactus, to be taken at the end of each meal. Chitosan (made from the shells of crustaceans) and Napol cactus bind ingested fat, preventing absorption, allowing it to be excreted in the stool. (Note: *You should not use this product if you have an allergy to shellfish.*)

While beneficial in the short term for losing weight, herbal combination supplements should be used in combination with the Naturopathic Diet and an exercise program. My recommendation is that natural weight-loss supplements be used periodically to help you through "plateau" phases in the diet, or on occasion, when faced with meals that fall outside your program.

Remember that these supplements are not needed for everyone on the Naturopathic Diet, and even when they are needed, supplements should be selected on an individual basis. As with any drug or natural supplement, we should inform our health care practitioner of its use.

Organic Food & Body Detoxification

ORGANIC FOOD & BODY DETOXIFICATION

While a great deal of our food is nutrient poor because of exhausted soils, processing, and storage, our food is also contaminated with chemical substances such as pesticides, herbicides, and growth hormones that not only impede weight loss but also jeopardize our general health. We need to choose 'clean' food and detoxify our body of contaminants if the Naturopathic Diet is to work effectively.

Certified Organic

There are a variety of terms used to describe 'healthy' food – organic, natural, and free range, for example. However, despite their widespread usage, there has been very little public education as to what they really mean. The term 'certified organic', whether it applies to livestock or fruits and vegetables, guarantees that no pesticides or hormones have gone into the growth of these foods. They are also guaranteed not to be genetically modified. With respect to animal products like meat and dairy, an organic label ensures no antibiotic use and a large area in which to run and live. There is a specific space requirement for each type of animal. If all these conditions are not met, then the animal is not considered organic.

With the emergence of organic foods and their growing popularity, other terms have appeared in an attempt to mimic the organic label or fool the consumer. Free range foods in general are cheaper than organic foods, and so when this label was born, many people unknowingly purchased these foods instead, thinking they were healthier. The term 'free-range' now means that animals have 'access' to the outdoors, but this encompasses everything from running chickens in a large field to housing 15,000 birds in a shed which has a gate that opens to the outside. More importantly, free-range animals are still fed on conventional pesticide-laden food. Similarly, they are routinely given antibiotics and growth hormone to increase production. So, we need to be very alert when we choose our food to ensure we will be eating organic food, free of these contaminants.

Growth Hormones

Insulin-like Growth Factor (IGF-1) was first synthesized in the 1980s and used as Bovine Growth Hormone to increase milk production in cows. It was so effective, yielding an average of 14% more milk when cows were injected every two weeks, that this procedure has now become standard. In 1985, the FDA (Food and Drug Administration) in the United States approved the sale of milk from injected cows and prohibited labeling on milk products that identified them as 'supplemented' with growth hormone.

IGF-1 is an important hormone produced in our liver and other body tissues. Human and bovine IGF-1 are structurally identical, making it very easy to interchange hormones between the two species. The production of IGF-1 is regulated by Human Growth Hormone (HGH), and its concentration in humans peaks at puberty and wanes throughout the rest of our lives.

IGF-1 is found in high concentration in the milk of cows who have been hormonally treated. The numbers show that treated cows have two to ten times the amount of IGF-1 in their milk. As well, the IGF-1 found in the milk of treated cows is much more potent than that found in regular cow's milk. This is because the IGF-1 in hormonally enhanced milk has a much greater affinity for other proteins in the body. The more strongly it binds, the more potent and long lasting the effect.

Human safety concerns have centered around the high levels of IGF-1 (Insulin-like Growth Factor) present in hormonally treated cow's milk. IGF-1 has been proven to stimulate the growth of normal cells, which is one reason why the agricultural community uses it. However, it has also known to stimulate the growth of cancerous cells. In several research studies, IGF-1 was observed to accelerate the growth of breast cancer and to contribute significantly to many childhood cancers, as well as small cell lung cancer, melanoma, and prostate cancer in adults. The most significant effect is on prostate cancer. IGF-1 level was found to be one of the most significant risk factors for prostate cancer. Men with levels between 300 and 500 ng/ml have greater than four times the risk of developing prostate cancer than men with levels around 100 to 185 ng/ml. The effects of IGF-1 also seem to become more threatening as men age. Men above 60 years of age had a risk of developing prostate cancer 8 times that of other men in the same age group if they had higher IGF-1 levels.

Further investigation into the absorption of IGF-1 is being carried out to determine whether IGF-1 is digested by enzymes, thereby negating any biological effect in humans. If IGF-1 is not broken down by enzymes, it will enter the intestine and be absorbed into the blood stream. Certainly, infants do not have the enzymes capable of breaking down this hormone until at least 6-9 months and are therefore at risk of absorption. Animal studies and human case studies have indicated that absorption does occur in adults. In addition, it is known that similar hormones such as Epidermal Growth Factor is not digested when mixed with casein, the main protein in milk.

Several countries, including Japan, Australia, and New Zealand, have now banned the use of bovine growth hormone. Until further investigation is completed and our cows are routinely spared hormone injections, the choice to ban these products from our diet is our choice. As individuals we can choose to drink and eat organic products available now in most stores.

Although IGF-1 can have detrimental effects in the body when it is too high, this hormone is also necessary for optimal health, metabolism, and weight loss. IGF-1 will bind to fat cells (adipocytes) and promote the release of their contained fat, thereby aiding the weight loss process. The blood level of this hormone may be screened through laboratory testing, and when abnormally low, can be increased effectively and safely though amino acid supplementation. In such a case, it is much safer to use the amino acids which act as precursors to IGF-1, and will aid the body in synthesizing more of its own IGF-1. When supplementing with amino acids, we can easily restore IGF-1 levels to normal and maximize the body's metabolism without increasing the levels above normal and increasing the risk of cancer. However, as most individuals have normal levels of this hormone, it is safer to avoid growth hormone in the diet.

Pesticide Exposure

Each day we are bombarded by pesticides in our food, in our water, and in the air we breathe. While these pesticides have decreased agricultural labor costs and increased crop production, they have placed our health at risk. More than 50 million kilograms of pesticides are used each year in Canada, with approximately 70% of this applied to crops and livestock food. The remaining 30% is allocated to forestry, gardening, indoor pest control, and golf course maintenance. Over 71 million pounds are used in the United States on home and garden use alone, and over 1.2 billion pounds of pesticide are used on American farms each year.

The term 'pesticide' encompasses herbicides, insecticides, and fungicides. There are on average approximately 600 active ingredients in these pesticides. Most pesticide formulations contain inert ingredients, compounds that assist in the transport of the active ingredient into the target pest. The active ingredient kills the pest.

Both inert and active ingredients can enter the human body. Pesticides may be inhaled, ingested in our food, or absorbed through the skin. Certain pesticides have been closely studied and have been linked to specific diseases or abnormalities. For example, one class of pesticide compounds known as organochlorines were studied by the Greater Boston Physicians for Social Responsibility and the Massachusetts Public Interest Research Group Education Fund, with the results published in the book *Generations at Risk: How Environmental Toxins May Affect Reproductive Health in Massachusetts*. These results were summarized in the following chart:

Pesticide Exposure

Organochlorine	Effect	Industrial Use
Lidane	decreases ovulation in rabbits	human lice tree farms
	testicular degeneration and androgen deficiency in rats	
Endosulfan	estrogen activity on breast tumors shrinks testicles in rats inhibits FSH and LH in rats decreased sperm count in mice	food application
Methoxychlor	estrogen activity blocked implantation and decreased fertility, and litter size in rats increased birth defects in rats	vegetables and fruits

Similar results were seen in another group of compounds called organophosphates.

Organophospate	Effect	Industrial Use
Parathion	DNA damage in rodents	fruits
Malathion	decreased progesterone in cows	fleas/tick control food
Diazanon	decreased sperm motility decreased testosterone increased fetal deaths and increased birth defects in mice	home use pesticides

Other epidemiological studies have been done indicating reproductive changes following occupational pesticide exposure to both men and women.

Occupation	Effect	Prevalence
Female Exposure		
Agriculture	spontaneous abortion	1.3 times more likely
Floriculture	spontaneous abortion	1.3 - 2.2 times more likely
	still births birth defects	
Male Exposure		
Agriculture	chromosomal abnormalities	30% more likely
Floriculture	chromosomal abnormalities	4 times more likely

Overall, this study and many others have concluded that pesticide exposure has reproductive and developmental consequences for human beings.

Other studies of the effect of pesticides found in groundwater in agricultural areas in the United States indicated significant effects on the nervous system, immune system, and endocrine system, specifically thyroid hormone. Thyroid hormone regulation and maintenance is essential for proper development of the brain prior to birth and during infancy. Some studies revealed ADD (Attention Deficit Disorder) and hyperactivity in children were linked to changes in thyroid hormone levels in the blood. Similarly, children with multiple chemical sensitivity had altered thyroid levels. As well, aggressive and irritable behavior was also linked to abnormal thyroid levels.

Although each pesticide has a different threshold of toxicity, children and infants are at highest risk. This is simply due to body weight. They are generally exposed to the same concentration of pesticide in the air and on food as most adults, yet they have substantially less body weight. Therefore, their relative concentration of pesticide per kilogram of body weight is much higher than an adult.

In another study, two different groups of children, aged four and five, controlled for socio-economic factors, were observed. One group had been continually exposed to pesticides as they lived on or near agricultural centers or farms. The other group lived on ranches with very little pesticide use. A decrease in mental and physical ability as well as an increase in aggression was seen in the children exposed to the pesticides. Those children who were routinely exposed to the pesticides displayed decreased hand-eye coordination and were unable to jump on the spot as long as those children who lived on the ranches. As well, the pesticide-exposed children were observed displaying more aggressive behavior to their siblings and were more emotionally labile. Overall changes in behavior and physical stamina were seen indicating changes in their immune, nervous, and endocrine systems.

Although further studies need to be done, preliminary reports do indicate that pesticides, even in low dose exposure, have many adverse effects on our body. We should do all that we can to eliminate our exposure and assist our bodies to detoxify. Without 'clean' food and a 'clean' body, the Naturopathic Diet will not be as effective and our long-term health will be jeopardized.

Body Detoxification

Although, to date, there is no clearly defined biochemical pathway to explain weight gain associated with a "toxic" body, we do know that a poorly nourished individual with high toxicity will not perform as well as a healthy one, especially with regard to weight loss. When the liver and kidneys are overworked, they neglect their regular duties such as glucose and fat metabolism and fluid control. Cellular energy is diverted into detoxification rather than exercise, growth, repair of tissue, immune control, and general well being. A 'clean' body will function better all round – and this can only aid weight loss and maintenance.

Kinds of Toxins

There are various types of toxins, but for simplicity, they can be categorized into three main groups. The first group of toxins are chemicals in the form of pesticides, drugs, and alcohol. These toxins primarily affect the liver and kidneys, the two main organs that must breakdown the pollutants and filter the blood. Symptoms of chemical toxicity are nausea, tingling in the extremities, jaundice, skin rashes, pruritis, and headaches.

The second group is heavy metals, such as cadmium, lead, arsenic, and aluminum. These metals accumulate as a result of direct exposure through the soil, cigarette smoke, contaminated fish, household cookware, tinned food, and other such environmental contaminants. These heavy metals are deposited in the bone and other tissues in the body, where they can create a wide variety of symptoms such as headaches, fatigue, muscle pain, decreased mental capabilities, pallor, and dizziness.

A third group of toxins are microbial in nature. This group would include gut bacteria and yeasts. Certain metabolic processes in the body, most notably those associated with attacking bacteria and viruses, also produce toxins. These toxins primarily affect the immune system, bowel, and skin, creating symptoms such as irritable bowel syndrome, ulcerative colitis, psorasis, and allergies.

The Detoxification Process

The body's main defense against such poisons takes place in the liver and kidneys. In reaction to pesticides, the liver begins to produce enzymes that breakdown the fat soluble chemicals. The detoxified products are then eliminated through the kidney, bowel, and skin. However, this is only possible for the pesticides that have been ingested. Pesticides or other chemicals that are inhaled through the lungs or absorbed through the skin are essentially free to roam the body, largely escaping liver detoxification.

Liver

The liver is a wedged shaped organ that lies beneath the rib cage in the upper right quadrant of the abdomen. Liver cells have the ability to regenerate following minimal damage. However, if there is injury or damage to the liver that exceeds its ability to regenerate, then there is a resulting decrease in liver function.

When toxin levels in the body increase, the liver must metabolize them (break them down into harmless and excreteable products). As this process requires energy, the liver must divert resources from its normal cellular activity like fat metabolism and recycling of cholesterol and other hormones. When this occurs, fat begins to build up within the liver, creating a condition known as fatty liver. Similarly, cholesterol is not broken down at its usual rate and blood levels consequently rise.

When the liver is overloaded and its normal functions impaired, symptoms such as malaise, nausea, and headaches occur along with clinical signs such as jaundice, skin eruptions, and itching. Blood levels of bilirubin (bile pigment) and liver enzymes may rise. In severe cases, liver failure may result.

Kidneys

The kidneys are two organs that lie adjacent to the aorta at the back of the abdomen, just to either side of the spine. These organs eliminate metabolic wastes, regulate electrolytes, influence the pH of the blood, and produce hormones such as prostaglandins and vitamin D. The kidneys must filter the blood of all its impurities. They can be somewhat likened to a sieve. Water mixed with a solid passing through the sieve may clog the holes. When this occurs, the rest of the water does not pass through readily and the holes in the sieve are temporarily damaged. While a sieve is unselective in what it filters out, the kidneys are highly specific. They can also actively reabsorb important chemicals, minerals, or electrolytes that are needed by the body. They can change the amounts or types of materials retained, depending on the overall state of the body's metabolism.

If the kidneys are damaged or the filters become clogged, then their function is decreased. This will result in less efficient filtration and toxin excretion and poorer resorption of important chemicals. Symptoms include fatigue, nausea, nocturia (having to get up to pass urine frequently at night), anorexia, and muscle twitching. In more advanced disease, hypertension, gastro-intestinal dysfunction, and mental slowing may occur.

Bowels, Skin, and Lungs

Although the kidney is the principal organ for excretion, the bowels, skin, and lungs also provide avenues for elimination of toxins or their metabolites. In the bowel, the colon acts as a temporary holding tank for the waste products. If these waste products linger for more than 24 hours, they begin to ferment from the gut bacteria and produce even more toxins. These toxins can then be reabsorbed back into the system, defeating the initial detoxification process. However, when the bowels are clearing daily, the majority of the toxins and waste by-products are eliminated in the stool.

Small amount of toxins are eliminated via sweat through the skin. An excess of toxins or poorly functioning skin and sweat glands can present as skin lesions, itchiness, and body odor. Almost any rash may be the result of a drug or toxin taken internally or applied to the skin.

The lungs provide one further source of excretion as long as the toxin can be carried in our breath. Bad breath is one obvious example of the effect of excessive toxins in our blood!

It is clear, therefore, that keeping these routes of elimination open and functioning optimally is crucial in ensuring that toxins do not build up in our body. But what do we do if, through diet, disease, or an unhealthy lifestyle, toxins begin to overload our system?

Detoxifying Techniques

There are a variety of herbs, supplements, and dietary programs that can be used to help detoxify the body. Not all are appropriate for everyone. Whenever an individual goes through a detoxification program, side effects can be seen. These sometimes include headaches, nausea, fatigue, and skin outbreaks. Accordingly, a detoxification program should be individually selected and monitored to minimize side effects and maximize results. When undergoing a detoxification program through the use of herbs, supplements, or pharmaceuticals, it is important to have it monitored by a health care practitioner. Some pre-existing conditions such as psorasis, cardiac conditions, bowel inflammatory conditions, and others may be aggravated and need to be accounted for prior to commencing any program. Although, in the long run, these conditions would benefit from detoxification, the program must be instituted more slowly to decrease any potential adverse reactions.

Several common herbs – milk thistle, tumeric, and dandelion, for example – are effective and safe for detoxification, as is the Naturopathic Diet itself.

Herbs

There are several herbs that can be used to help repair inflammation, protect liver cells, and regenerate them. The first is Milk Thistle or *Silymarin marianum*. This herb has hepatoreparative and hepatoprotective properties achieved through stimulation of RNA polymerase and DNA synthesis. Simply put, this herb helps to protect the healthy cells in the liver from harm or inflammation as well as stimulate the regeneration of new healthy cells. As this occurs, the liver is able to function more effectively. Milk thistle also competes for toxin binding sites with alpha-amonitin and phalloidoin and therefore aids the body in mopping up toxins. This herb has no adverse side effects, though it may loosen stools slightly as it increases bile flow.

Another herb that can be used is Tumeric or *Curcuma longa*. This herb has been shown to have anti-inflammatory activity comparable to that of hydrocortisone and phenylbutazone. Furthermore, tumeric is thought to inhibit cortisone metabolism in the liver, thereby increasing circulating cortisone. Tumeric increases the breakdown of fibrin, promotes increased liver function, increases bile flow, and protects the liver from incoming toxins. This herb essentially has no adverse side effects, although in some individuals it may irritate the gastro intestinal tract with prolonged chronic use. Like milk thistle, this herb may soften stools due to the increase in bile flow.

Yet another herb that can be used to help detoxify the body is Dandelion or *Taraxacum officinalis*. This herb acts upon both the kidneys and the liver. Although its mechanism is not thoroughly understood, dandelion has diuretic properties. It is known to have potassium sparing effects, which most diuretics do not have.

Similarly, the saponins that exist in dandelion are thought to degrade mucopolysaccharide foci (components in kidney stones) and therefore help to protect the kidney against stones.

Dandelion's liver action lies in its choleretic properties (increasing bile production) and its cholagogue properties (increasing the contraction of the bile duct to release the stored bile). Despite its benefits, dandelion may have some adverse reactions in some people. Contact dermatitis has been seen when the herb is used in fresh form rather than dried. As well, if an occluded bile duct is present, this herb should not be administered.

The Naturopathic Diet

We are often unable to change toxic factors such as the air we breathe (beyond not exercising during rush hour traffic!), but we can change our diet. By eliminating the simple sugars, alcohol, caffeine, additives, and preservatives in our diet, we will automatically lessen the load on the liver. This, in turn, will begin the detoxification process. From here, we can choose organic foods to decrease our exposure to pesticides and hormones; and we can choose foods that will stimulate the cleansing or detoxification process in the liver by stimulating the production of extra enzymes that break down those toxins. These foods include lemons, beets, carrots, and artichokes. By increasing the consumption of these foods – by beginning the day with hot water and lemon instead of coffee, for example – we can stimulate the liver to function at its maximum capacity.

The value of the Naturopathic Diet is thus manifold. Not only do we lose weight quickly and maintain weight loss permanently, we detoxify our bodies and help prevent disease.

Soy Food Proteins & Phytoestrogens

Beneficial Hormonal Effects
Anti-Cancer Properties
Lower Cholesterol
Varieties of Soy Food

SOY FOOD PROTEINS
& PHYTOESTROGENS

S oy food has always been abundantly used in the Eastern diet, but in the Western world, 'soy' for may years only referred to a salty sauce prepared from the soybean to compliment fish, meat, rice, and 'oriental' dishes. Soybean seed oil was also used for cooking and storing foods. We now generally refer to soy as any product made from the soybean, including tofu and misso. Only recently have these protein rich soy foods become popular in Western diets. For the Naturopathic Diet, soy foods are highly recommended, not only as a good source of protein, but also as a source of phytoestrogens, which have a valuable role in balancing our hormones and fighting cancer and other diseases.

The soybean is a leguminous plant. All soybean products, such as tofu or misso, are complete proteins, containing all the required amino acids for daily living. This is particularly important for the vegetarian, for there are very few vegetarian sources that are complete proteins. Most other vegetarian protein sources, like nuts and other beans, are incomplete and must be supplemented in the vegetarian diet.

In addition to its function as a protein source, soy is now being recognized for its numerous therapeutic properties, such as lowering cholesterol, preventing and aiding in the treatment of cancer, minimizing menstrual and menopausal symptoms as well as governing menstrual irregularities. Soy is also used in a variety of other chronic conditions.

Beneficial Hormonal Effects

S oybeans contain several active ingredients, including protease inhibitors, phytosterols or isoflavones, and saponins. The constituents drawing the most attention are the isoflavones. Two particular isoflavones have been studied extensively: genistein and daidzin. They have been found to be beneficial in the treatment of hormonal disorders, cancer, and hypercholesterolemia.

Phytosterols are plant chemicals that are structurally very similar to the endogenous hormones produced in our bodies. The main phytosterols investigated in soy are phytoestrogens or plant estrogens. These phytoestrogens are so similar to our own estrogen that they will bind into the same receptors in our body that our own naturally occurring estrogen does. This in turn produces an estrogenic effect. In order for a hormone to be active or produce any effect in the body, it must bind into a receptor. This is its site of action. If it does not bind into this spot, no therapeutic or metabolic reaction will occur. Thus, if these phytosterols were not structurally similar to our own hormones, they would not fit into these receptors and would not have an effect. Receptors are very specific. They will only allow or accept an equally specific structure to bind. This receptor specificity becomes a very important factor when searching for natural foods or supplements that will have a therapeutic effect on the body. Soy, and its phytosterols, are specific enough to allow this reaction to take place.

Isoflavones are the most common type of phytoestrogens and structurally resemble estrogen. However, they have the ability to act as an estrogen *or* an anti-estrogen. Phytoestrogens or isoflavones possess both an estrogenic and anti-estrogenic quality, depending on how they are used and in which type of individual. It is partially through the manipulation of this dual property that isoflavones have their therapeutic effect.

If an individual is deficient in estrogen, for example, as occurs in menopause, proper supplementation with isoflavones will increase the amount of estrogen-like activity in the body, thereby alleviating the menopausal symptoms. Isoflavones are much weaker, possessing from 1/1000 to 1/100000 the activity of endogenous estrogen, and will therefore have a smaller or weaker effect, but with proper supplementation, the effect that they produce is large enough to reduce or cease menopausal symptoms but too small to induce a period in most women.

It is this 'weak' property of isoflavones that also gives them their anti-estrogen effect. If one has higher levels of estrogen, as seen in polycystic ovary syndrome, endometriosis, or excessive pre-menstrual syndrome, phytoestrogens or isoflavones can help to lower the amount of effective estrogen in the body. This again is due to the structural similarity. The isoflavones compete with our own estrogen for the receptor or binding sites in the body. When an isoflavone binds into a receptor, it blocks the site at which a stronger estrogen may bind. Thus a weaker form of estrogen fills the receptor, lowering the overall activity of estrogen in the body.

This mechanism becomes particularly useful when treating hormonally related disorders. During menopause the production of estrogen drops greatly, which can trigger a variety of different symptoms, from hot flashes and sweats to insomnia and vaginal dryness. According to life expectancy figures, most women will live one-third of their lives in this menopausal or lowered hormonal state. Several studies have now demonstrated that a statistically significant reduction in hot flashes, vaginal dryness, anxiety, and insomnia can be achieved through the addition of isoflavones to the diet of menopausal women. Approximately 80 mg of isoflavones a day yielded a 45% reduction in symptoms reported by 104 women in a study conducted in Belgium. This is also demonstrated in a review in the *Canadian Family Physician* stating that phytoestrogens play a substantial role in diminishing menopausal symptoms and possibly protect against cardiovascular disease and bones loss.

Conversely, phytoestrogens are used to lower the amount of effective estrogen in those people who have higher levels or an imbalance of estrogen to progesterone. In the symptomatic menstruating female with high estrogen levels, cramps, bloating, and heavy bleeding are well-known symptoms. Through the supplementation of a weaker form of estrogen (isoflavones), the amount of estrogenic activity is lowered by blocking the estrogen receptors. In doing so, the stronger endogenous estrogen can no longer bind and the clinical symptoms are greatly improved. The same holds true for almost any estrogen related symptom or disorder.

Anti-Cancer Properties

One in nine women in North America will develop breast cancer; however, women in Southeast Asia whose diets are rich in soy (approximately 10-50 grams/day) are four to six times less likely to develop breast cancer. Genetic differences have failed to explain this dramatic reduction in risk. While the soy-related lowering of estrogen levels appears to decrease the risk of developing certain estrogen receptor cancers such as breast cancer, there seems to be another factor involved. Soy also decreases cancer formation and growth by inhibiting tumor cell differentiation. Cell differentiation is the process of cell division from an immature state to its final destined mature cell type. If the destiny of an immature cell can be controlled so that it does not form into a cancerous cell, the therapeutic benefits of soy could be outstanding.

Modification of cellular growth and differentiation is achieved through the control of the enzyme tyrosine kinase. Studies have implicated increased activity of tyrosine kinase in many different cancers. Trials have continually proven that the isoflavone genistein is able to inhibit the activity of tyrosine kinase, thereby aiding in the treatment and prevention of cancer. Furthermore, genistein has been shown to inhibit TOPO (DNA Topoisomerase). This is one of the principal enzymes involved in DNA replication and transcription. Many of the anti-tumor products used in chemotherapy today are directed at inhibiting TOPO.

Soy appears to be a noteworthy supplement in the treatment of cancer. A summary of 861 studies collected between the years of 1980 to 1995 revealed that phytoestrogens play a beneficial role in protecting not only against breast cancer but also prostate, colon, rectal, stomach, and lung cancer. This is accounted for by both the anti-estrogenic properties and the inhibition of cancer growth and formation.

More recent studies have revealed that another isoflavone, daidzin, also contains a valuable therapeutic effect. When consumed in high concentration (approximately 20-40 mg/kg of body weight), daidzin had a nonspecific immune stimulatory effect in mice. This response was not observed at lower levels of daidzin, such as 10 mg/kg of body weight. This non-specific reaction includes increased phagocytotic activity and an increased number of available macrophages. Phagocytosis is the ingestion of micro-organisms, cells, and foreign particles. Macrophages are large phagocytic cells found in many tissues. They play an important role in the clearance of inflammatory cells and other debris. Thus macrophages and phagacytes are part of the body's cleansing apparatus, removing unwanted debris that can contribute to disease.

Lower Cholesterol

Hypercholesterolemia is another prevalent disease that can be treated in part through the Naturopathic Diet. A diet rich in soy food supplements this benefit. Soy plays a dual role in this process. First, it is an excellent protein source and an integral part of the diet. This in itself can have a dramatic effect on the level of cholesterol and fats in the blood. Second, isoflavones alone have been shown to reduce cholesterol levels significantly. In one study by the American Heart Association, a 10% reduction in both total cholesterol and LDLs was observed after just 9 weeks of isoflavone supplementation. A dose-dependant relationship was also discovered when four groups, each receiving different isoflavone supplementation levels, were compared. The concentrations used were 4 mg, 25 mgs, 42 mg, and 58 mg of isoflavones per day. As the amount of isoflavone concentration increased, a greater reduction in total cholesterol and LDLs was observed.

Genistein has been shown to have another beneficial affect with respect to cholesterol. Studies have found genistein to be a potent antioxidant in both fat or lipophilic tissue and water-soluble environments. Thus genistein increases the resistance of LDL to oxidation and subsequently arterial damage. As we age, the elasticity or stretching capacity of our blood vessels decreases. This is yet another contributing factor to high blood pressure and heart disease. Supplementation with 45 mg of genistein or 80 mg of isoflavone over a 10-week period significantly improved arterial compliance or vessel elasticity. Soy isoflavones had as beneficial an effect on arterial health as conventional hormone replacement therapy. Isoflavones not only play an integral role in cholesterol reduction, but also in the subsequent treatment of heart disease and arteriosclerosis.

Can you have too much of a good thing? Is there a possibility that phytoestrogens can have a negative or adverse effect on the body? Although more investigation on this topic needs to be done, it holds true that anything, whether it is a plant or a pharmaceutical drug, can have a detrimental affect if it can have a positive one. Due to the fact that there are actual biochemical and endocrine changes that take place with isoflavone supplementation, it would make sense that too much could be harmful. While consultation with your health care practitioner is recommended before treatment of any of these conditions, it would appear that soy, in regular dietary amounts, is perfectly safe.

Varieties of Soy Food

The amount of active therapeutic ingredient in soy food varies greatly. The isoflavone genistein, one of the main elements in soy, is more readily available in fermented soy products like misso or natto. This is because of the B-glycosyl bond that occurs in genstein, the precursor to genestein. This bond is broken to form excess genistein during the fermentation process, therefore yielding a higher concentration of active ingredient.

The following chart displays different soybean products and their corresponding genistein concentrations.

Varieties of Soy Food

Product	microgram (mcg) Genistein per gram (g) food
Soy Nuts	4.6-8.2
Soy Powder	200-961
Soy Milk	1.9-13.9
Tofu	94.8-137.7
Misso	38.5-229.1
Natto	71.7-492.8

As can be seen from this chart, there is a slight variation in genistein content even within each food type. This is accounted for by small differences in food types within one particular soy product group. For example, tofu is available in many different forms. The soybean protein composition of tofu and other soy products is generally related to the texture, although it must be noted that this is not universal across all soy products. In general, the firmer the tofu, the higher the protein content and the lower the fat concentration.

Many of these soy foods are now available in organic form at our local chain grocery stores, no longer consigned only to health food stores.

The Naturopathic Diet
for Children

Children's Metabolism
Retraining a Child's Metabolism
Children's Protein Needs
Children's Attitude Towards Food
Exercise
Children and Pesticides

THE NATUROPATHIC DIET
FOR CHILDREN

Why do children's diets need special attention? They seem to be little adults – they get hungry, they put on weight, just like us. There are, however, some important differences between children and adults that make them deserving of special dietary care.

Most important is the fact that children are still growing and developing. They are laying down the foundations of a body that needs to last them the rest of their lives. Like the fable of the three little pigs, if we build a house of straw, it will fall in the slightest breeze, yet a house of brick can withstand the many onslaughts of the world around us. If we feed a growing body poor building materials – foods that are nutrient-scarce or a poorly balanced diet – the child's body will be less likely to grow strong and will lack day-to-day endurance, with little resistance to infection or disease.

As with adults, children's food is their fuel, but in a child, every cell is growing and multiplying at a faster rate. What children eat early in their development sets the metabolic stage for their future weight, fat deposition, muscle bulk, and ability to handle a more diverse diet. While adults still require protein and other nutrients to repair damaged tissue and to account for daily turnover, the child's requirements are substantially higher when size is accounted for.

With children, it is important to differentiate between normal, healthy weight gain associated with growth and unhealthy gain associated with obesity and metabolic abnormality. Childhood obesity is reaching epidemic proportions. This abnormal type of weight gain is typified by the development of fat deposits around the midsection. These deposits are generally softer and "puffier" than healthy tissue. To determine a healthy weight for your child, reference to weight and growth percentile charts for height and age will give useful information as to your child's status.

For children, nutrition influences not only their weight and physical development. It also affects their emotional moods and sleep patterns as well as their ability to learn. A poor diet plays a role in attention deficit disorders (ADD). And like adults, a child's diet can contribute to disease conditions, specifically non-insulin-dependant diabetes and high cholesterol. Like obesity, these 'adult' diseases have become near epidemic in proportion among children. If we truly care about our children's welfare, the greatest gift we can give them is a sound nutritional foundation.

Children's Metabolism

Children's metabolism is similar to that of adults in terms of hormonal output. They secrete insulin when they eat too many sugars, grains, and starches. They also store excess carbohydrate as fat, over-secrete insulin, and decrease the use of their food as fuel. How they differ from adults relates to the amount of hormonal output and the plasticity of their metabolic pathways.

As with adults, whenever grains and starches are ingested by children blood sugars rise very quickly through the rapid breakdown of these foods into sugar. This raises the blood sugar level above normal and forces the pancreas to secrete insulin, our storage hormone. Insulin then sweeps this excess sugar out of the blood and stores it, initially as glycogen (our limited sugar stores) and then as fat. Over time, the more meals we consume that are rich in grains and starches and devoid of protein, the more insulin is required to cope with the rising sugar levels. This leads to the state of hyperinsulinemia, and ongoing hyper-secretion of insulin blocks the use of fat as a fuel source, forcing the body to default to muscle as an alternative.

Children are just a susceptible to hyperinsulinemia as adults but generally have not had as many years for this condition to develop. Children who have not yet reached their insulin threshold may maintain a relatively stable weight despite consuming vast amounts of sugar, pop, pasta, and bread, but if this pattern remains unchanged and they are not taught to balance their meals with protein, the majority will progress towards the metabolic 'mess' that afflicts 76% of our North American population.

The statistics on the increase in childhood obesity, cardiovascular disease, and diabetes are frightening. In the United States, there has been a 54% rise in childhood obesity since the 1960s, as reported in the *Journal of Disease of Children*. A 1998 article published in the *Journal of the American Medical Association* currently reveals that childhood obesity in the United States afflicts approximately 25% of all children. Studies performed in the United Kingdom show a rise in childhood obesity from 5% to 19% from 1984 to 1994. Among overweight children aged 5-15 years, 61% already have one or more cardiovascular risk factors, while 27% of them have two or more, as reported in the *British Medical Journal* in 2000. The *Journal of the American Academy of Pediatrics* in March 2000 published a study showing that childhood Type-2 diabetes in on the rise. In 1990, less than 4% of children aged 10 to 19 were diagnosed with this condition. Those numbers have risen approximately 20% in the last 10 years. Of those children diagnosed with Type-2 diabetes, a staggering 85% of them were clinically obese.

Some unfortunate children have the additional disadvantage of being born with a metabolism already primed for hyperinsulinemia. Not only will they have inherited a genetic predisposition to hyper-secrete insulin from their parents, but a poor maternal diet during pregnancy will also have pre-programmed the infant's metabolic and hormonal pathways. These children often start life on the chubby side and retain a tendency to gain weight throughout childhood and into adult life. Mothers, if your child has these tendencies, take a look back to how you ate prior to and during pregnancy. Did you start your pregnancy a little heavier than you would have wished, were you consuming a great deal of carbohydrate to help combat nausea, or was your pregnancy weight gain higher than average? If you answered yes to any of those questions, then there is a strong possibility that your child's metabolism may be more sensitive to sugars, grains, and starches, making it easier for your child to pack on the pounds.

Retraining a Child's Metabolism

Fortunately, the undesirable effects of hyperinsulinemia can be prevented and reversed in children, just as they can in adults. The good news is that it does not usually take as long. Even though children may be secreting more insulin than they should after a bagel or pasta meal, they have not had years and years of this dietary assault. The metabolic abnormalities are therefore not quite as ingrained or imprinted as those of an adult. In addition, the overall amount of insulin secreted is usually less. They have not escalated their production to the extremes seen in an adult who has consumed many more carbohydrate-dominant meals. Because of these factors, it generally takes less time for a child to reverse the entire process. For example, a child may not have to spend eight weeks in the first stage of the Naturopathic Diet before moving on to the maintenance stage.

Stage One: Weight Loss

Because every child is different, it is important to look for the signs of hyperinsulinemia. The extent to which children display these signs will indicate to us how hyperinsulinemic they are. Have they already reached that threshold, or are they still storing the normal amount of sugar as fat through lower hormonal output?

To review the signs of hyperinsulinemia, we are looking for symptoms that indicate a high level of insulin secretion following a meal. Immediate signs will be fatigue as the sugar, which was supposed to be providing fuel for your child's body, is swept out of the blood. This will make them tired or irritable. As in an adult, they may feel bloated after the meal, complaining of abdominal fullness or discomfort.

The degree to which these symptoms appear is used to determine how long a child is required to stay in the weight loss stage of the Naturopathic Diet before moving on to the maintenance stage. To determine this degree, I divide children into three categories. If the symptoms rarely appear, or appear only following a particularly starchy or sugar-rich meal, and the child has not shown a weight-gain tendency, secretion of insulin is essentially normal. These children I classify as *Category 1*. If they have these symptoms following all meals of predominantly pasta, breads, grains, or cereal, with little to no protein, and have gained only a small amount of weight, then they most likely are beginning to secrete a higher than normal amount of insulin after these meals. These children belong in *Category 2*. If, however, they feel bloated and tired following most meals, and are displaying puffy central weight gain, then they are definitely secreting high levels of insulin after each meal and storing more than normal amounts of fat. These children I place in *Category 3*.

Category 1:

This category is for those children who have not yet taught their metabolisms to secrete high levels of insulin. They are responding quite normally to most meals and have not yet gained extra weight, particularly around the central trunk area. In addition, they do not appear to be sleepy or bloated following a meal. It is normal for a child or an adult to get nervous, excited, or overly energized following a large intake of sugar. This is usually accompanied by a "crash" or overwhelming fatigue 20-40 minutes later. This is not necessarily representative of hyperinsulinemia. However, if you allow your child to experience this roller-coaster continually, then their metabolism will soon learn that it needs to secrete more than the normal amount of insulin to cope with the dietary intake of sugar.

This is the easiest stage to reverse and then establish healthy metabolic pathways, as the child is still within normal limits to begin with. It only takes a short period of time to teach the body to 'cue' into protein rather than carbohydrate at each meal. For this reason, a child in Category 1 would follow the same diet as an adult in stage one of the Naturopathic Diet. The child would only have to follow it for two weeks. This would be sufficient time to retrain a Category 1 child's metabolism and ensure that a healthy metabolic state was achieved before entering the maintenance stage.

Category 2:

This category is for those children who have already started to develop a hyperinsulinemic tendency. They are already displaying the signs of this metabolic state, such as mild weight gain, fatigue, bloating after meals high in carbohydrates, and possibly irritability and loss of concentration. They have not, however, reached their insulin threshold. If they have a meal that is balanced with protein, then their energy remains normal to high with no "crash". This is the child who loves breads, cereals, and pastas, but is only asking for them at meal times.

Reversal for Category 2 still does not require as much time in stage one of the Naturopathic Diet as for an adult or a child in Category 3. It does take more time than a child in Category 1 because a Category 2 child is further along the course of metabolic deterioration and therefore requires more time to retrain the pathways back to normal. A Category 2 child should remain in stage one for four weeks. Following this, the child can go straight into the maintenance stage, again watching for hyperinsulinemic signs as grains, starches, and sugars are re-introduced just to ensure that the child's metabolism has altered back to normal.

To review this re-introduction procedure: Upon re-introduction of the forbidden carbohydrates for either a child in Category 2 or 3 or an adult, it is important to make sure that the insulin metabolism has completely reversed before entering the maintenance stage permanently. If the insulin secretion has not quite altered itself, then the same hyperinsulinemic signs will be seen upon carbohydrate ingestion, even when combined with protein. These signs will be less, so careful attention is needed. If the signs are still present, then return to the weight loss stage for one week. After this week, try to re-introduce the grains and starches again, and then look for the bloating and fatigue signs following their ingestion. Once you find that they no longer occur, move permanently into the maintenance stage of the Naturopathic Diet without any fear of regaining weight or altering metabolism.

Category 3:

Children in Category 3 have consumed many meals rich in carbohydrate and devoid of protein. They have taught their body, much like an adult, to hypersecrete insulin following each meal. They are therefore storing a lot of their food as fat and will be gaining more than normal amounts of weight for a growing child. Similarly, they most likely will be bloated following most meals (complaints of abdominal fullness or discomfort), and they will be tired and irritable. Their level of concentration, particularly after meals, will be poor, and this may affect their learning ability. These children are at a high risk for obesity and diabetes, with the prospect of a lifetime of dieting. However, they too can reverse this process and enjoy normal eating patterns, avoid weight gain and reduce their lifetime risk of disease.

To reverse the metabolism of Category 3 children will require almost as much time as for an adult. It usually takes six weeks of stage one of the Naturopathic Diet to retrain the body of a child in Category 3 back to normal. Once again, when the child enters the maintenance stage, it is important to watch for the hyperinsulinemic signs to ensure that the metabolic alteration is complete. As long as there are no symptoms of the hyperinsulinemia, then your child may remain in the maintenance stage indefinitely.

Summary

	Central "puffy" weight gain	Fatigue	Bloating	Mood change	Time spent in Stage 1
Category 1	No	No	No	No	2 weeks
Category 2	Mild	Yes	Mild	Yes	4 weeks
Category 3	Marked	Yes	Yes	Yes	6 weeks

Children's Protein Needs

As with adults, the amount of protein that a child should consume each day is dependant on many factors. The most important factor is size. Due to the fact that children are still growing, and every cell in their body requires protein to reproduce, children actually require a higher ratio of protein to body weight than adults do. For a sedentary child, 1 to 1.2 grams of protein per kilogram of body weight is what they need to stabilize blood sugar levels, replace and repair muscle, produce antibodies, and regulate hormones. If a child is particularly active (frequent, competitive exercise, for example), more protein will be needed to repair the continual breakdown of muscle and will require production of more hormones, antibodies, and enzymes due to the increased demand. This child should consume 1.2 to 1.5 grams of protein per kilogram of body weight. So, a 60-pound, or 27-kilogram child, doing little exercise, should be consuming 27 to 33 grams of protein a day. This protein should not be all in one sitting, but rather spread out across meals, roughly 10 grams of protein per meal. (See charts for food equivalents.) If the child is active, participating in sports for one or more hours a day, 33 to 41 grams of protein should be consumed each day.

By following these simple rules, it is very easy to re-establish healthy metabolic function. This in turn will allow your child to enjoy a wide variety of foods without concern over health or weight, and, more importantly, without increasing the risk of heart disease, diabetes, high cholesterol, and obesity.

As with an adult, the same issues surrounding protein intake apply. If a child has a pre-existing disease or does not have full kidney function, then the amount of protein changes. In these cases, it is recommended that you discuss the diet with your health care practitioner to establish the correct balance for your individual child. If your child is generally healthy and free of disease, there is no need for concern about protein consumption. Just as a pregnant mother requires more than the average intake of protein to allow the baby inside her to grow, so does a child. Although our bodies may stop growing in terms of height in our teens or early twenties, it is not until our late twenties and early thirties that we enter "our transitional years." It is during these years that our bodies technically stop growing and start aging. This is where the rate of cellular turn declines and we therefore require fewer calories and less food to sustain our bodies. These recommendations can, therefore, be followed from early childhood through adolescence into early adult life.

Protein Needs for Stage 1 and 2	
Less active child	1.0 - 1.2 grams per kilogram body weight
More active child	1.2 - 1.5 grams per kilogram body weight

Children's Attitude Towards Food

If we establish healthy eating patterns and encourage sound food choices for our children early in their lives, they will not only live a life relatively free of many diseases, but they will never struggle with the weight issues that plague our generation. They will develop a healthy attitude towards their food. We need to teach our children that the Naturopathic Diet is not a fad 'diet' or 'pop' weight loss program to improve their body image. While the Naturopathic Diet will enable weight loss and prevent obesity, the aim is to establish the foundation for lifelong good health, not to sculpt the body to match fashion trends.

The food choices for children are as varied as they are for adults in stage one of the Naturopathic Diet. Children need a sufficient amount of carbohydrate, particularly during stage one. They can consume an unlimited amount of vegetables and salads. They can use any condiment or dressing they like. Just like the adults, children should only have two fruits a day, and no bananas.

We should encourage children to eat vegetables. In our society where nutrient-poor foods are forcefully advertised, children do not naturally gravitate towards healthy vegetables, so try to make them fun by using dips and spices. As children require more calories per pound of body weight than an adult, we have more room to "play" with in terms of fat. They can have more cheese and dips than adults without being too concerned about the fat content, especially as many fats have been eliminated through avoidance of candy, bagels, cookies, and other carbohydrates. An example of this would be low fat yogurt mixed with an onion soup mix as a dip for carrots, celery, and peppers. To make cooked vegetables more exciting, try melting cheddar cheese and mixing it with cottage cheese and pouring it over steamed broccoli and green beans (see Recipes & Menus chapter for these and other ideas).

Exercise

A change in lifestyle over the past few decades has also greatly contributed to childhood obesity and diabetes. There has been a significant reduction in energy expenditure as more and more children spent their time playing computer games and watching television more and more. In the past, most children would play actively outside after school or participate in a sport. More often than not, children in today's society rush home to sit at their desk to use the PC or slouch in front of the television. A decrease in exercise not only reduces the number of calories burned, it will decrease muscle mass and therefore fat burning potential. In addition, most children snack while watching television, enticed by the advertisements for fast and fried foods. This learned behavior, often copied from parents, will follow the child into adulthood and therefore perpetuate what is an important component of an unhealthy lifestyle. As a complement to the Naturopathic Diet, encourage your children to exercise.

Children and Pesticides

Another area of concern with our children's diet is that of pesticides on our food and chemicals in our food containers. Each day we are bombarded with pesticides in our food, in our water, and in the air we breathe. While these pesticides have decreased agricultural labor costs and increased crop production, they have placed our health at risk. More than 50 million kilograms of pesticides are used each year in Canada, with approximately 70% of this applied to crops and livestock food. The remaining 30% is allocated to forestry, gardening, indoor pest control, and golf course maintenance. Over 71 million pounds are used in the United States on home and garden use alone, and over 1.2 billion pounds of pesticide are used on American farms each year.

The term 'pesticide' encompasses herbicides, insecticides, and fungicides. There are, on average, approximately 600 active ingredients in these pesticides. Most pesticide formulations contain both inert and active ingredients. Inert compounds assist in the transport of the active ingredient into the target pest. The active ingredient then kills the pest. Both inert and active ingredients can enter the human body. Pesticides may be inhaled, ingested in our food, or absorbed through the skin. Certain pesticides have been linked to specific diseases or abnormalities. Some of these are discussed in the Organic Food & Body Detoxification chapter.

Although each pesticide has a different threshold of toxicity, children and infants are at highest risk. This is simply due to body weight. They are generally exposed to the same concentration of pesticide in the air and on food as most adults, yet they have substantially less body weight. Therefore, their relative concentration of pesticide per kilogram of body weight is much higher than an adult.

With specific reference to children, some studies on the effects of pesticides found in groundwater in agricultural areas in the United States indicated significant effects on the nervous system, immune system, and endocrine system, specifically thyroid hormone. Thyroid hormone regulation and maintenance is essential for proper development of the brain prior to and immediately following birth. Some studies reveal that ADD (Attention Deficit Disorder) and hyperactivity in children, including aggressive and irritable behavior, are linked to changes in thyroid hormone levels in the blood.

In another study, two different groups of children, aged four and five, controlled for socio-economic factors, were observed. One group had been continually exposed to pesticides because they lived on or near agricultural centers or farms. The other group lived on ranches with very little pesticide use. A decrease in mental and physical ability as well as an increase in aggression was seen in the children exposed to the pesticides. Those children who were routinely exposed to the pesticides displayed decreased hand-eye coordination and were unable to jump on the spot as long as those children who lived on the ranches. As well, the pesticide-exposed children were observed displaying more aggressive behavior to their siblings and were more emotionally labile. Overall changes in behavior and physical stamina were seen, indicating changes in their immune, nervous, and endocrine systems.

Precocious puberty, or early onset of puberty, has increased greatly over the past few decades. Studies have demonstrated a direct link between chemicals in the environment and early maturation in females. In one such study carried out in the United States, reported by the Environmental News Network in 2001, 17,000 female children were observed for early onset of sexual development: 15% of Caucasian girls in the study and 48% of African-Americans started to develop breasts and pubic hair by eight years of age. Some of these children began sexual development as early as two years old. As reported in a 2001 issue of the journal *Human Reproduction*, similar studies conducted in Belgium around developing areas, where the chemical exposure was greater, revealed a larger number of children with precocious puberty. Of great importance was that most of them had consistently higher levels of DDT metabolites in their blood plasma samples.

Further research on mice has revealed the dangers of chemicals that can leach out of food containers into our food and water. BPA, or bisphenol A, is a chemical used in manufacturing many plastic products such as baby bottles, water bottles, tin can linings, certain plastic toys, and some food storage containers. This chemical leaches out of the plastic and into the food, water, or substrate that it touches. The rate at which BPA leaks increases with continued use of the plastic product. BPA has been shown to mimic estrogen. For that reason, it is referred to as an endocrine disrupter that can disrupt the delicate hormonal balance in the body. As reported in BBC News Science and Technology, scientists at of University of Missouri-Columbia and North Carolina State University investigated the effects of BPA on mice. They discovered that when pregnant mice were exposed to BPA, their offspring weighed 20% more at puberty. Similarly, the mice showed premature puberty. Scientists now believe that this chemical exposure over the past few decades, both *in utero* and early on in life, may be a large contributing factor to the changing hormonal and reproductive trends seen in the human population today.

These, and many other studies, are of great concern to the health and welfare of our children. We are silently altering their reproductive systems and influencing growth and weight gain. Of even more concern is the possible risk of cancer from the direct, early onset of estrogen exposure. We have known for a very long time that the risk of developing breast cancer, an estrogenic receptor dependent cancer, increases when a woman has early onset of menses and late onset menopause. This is simply due to an increase in the number of years that she is exposed to estrogen. With precocious puberty on the rise, our children are at even greater risk than we are as adults.

Once again, the majority of this risk may be diminished through the use of organic produce and non-plastic food containers, combined with the principles of the Naturopathic Diet.

Frequently Asked Questions about the Naturopathic Diet

Frequently Asked Questions about the Naturopathic Diet

1. Do I have to stay off grains and starches forever?

NO! You must refrain from grains, starches and sugars for a minimum of eight weeks (Stage One of the diet). This time period is required to retrain the body's metabolism such that when you do reintroduce those carbohydrates, you do not store them as fat. Once this initial eight-week period is finished, it is up to you whether or not to begin reintroducing them. As soon as you bring them in on a daily basis, the weight loss process halts. As long as they are combined properly with protein (as described in this book), weight will not be regained.

If you wish to continue to lose more weight after the initial eight-week period, you simply remain in stage one for longer. Once you have achieved your goal weight, you may progress to stage two and return to eating grains and starches daily at the appropriate proportion and combination. You do not have to eliminate grains and starches forever, only temporarily.

2. Will I gain the weight back when I reintroduce carbohydrates?

NO! Once metabolism has been reset from the first eight weeks of the diet, it is now tuned to recognize protein first and break the incoming food down slowly. This means that the blood sugar levels do not rise quickly and insulin is not released at a high rate. If insulin is not released at a high rate, then the carbohydrate will not be stored as fat.

When reintroducing carbohydrates, it is important to follow the guidelines described in the book. The grain and starch reintroduction must happen slowly, and those carbohydrates must be consumed at the same time as protein. The same philosophy applies when reintroducing other carbohydrates. As long as insulin is not released at a high rate, then the incoming food will still not be stored as fat and weight gain will not occur. When grains and starches are reintroduced, insulin levels will rise slightly. This is what stops further weight loss. However, as long as that rise in insulin is kept to a minimum, the weight gain will not occur. The rise is kept to a minimum by combining those grains and starches with protein.

As long as you stick to the rule where the physical amount of protein is greater than or equal to the amount of carbohydrate, this metabolic balance will remain, and so will your weight loss.

3. Will this diet harm my kidneys?

NO! This diet will not injure, inflame, or harm the kidneys in any way.

Renal (or kidney) damage occurs when a condition called ketosis is induced. Continual protein in high concentration by itself, without any carbohydrate, will stimulate ketosis, a starvation state in which the insulin and glucose levels are very low and glucagon levels rise. The liver produces a small amount of glucose and significant amounts of ketone bodies. All tissues can use ketones as fuel, and this helps prevent excess protein breakdown during prolonged starvation, but this state is unhealthy for the body, particularly the kidneys, so should be avoided. This is why we must add carbohydrates to the meal.

Ketosis only occurs when there is too much protein and not enough carbohydrate in the diet. Some diets actually try to induce this condition as it results in rapid, but not permanent, weight loss. In a ketotic diet, the amount of carbohydrate consumed per meal is approximately 5 to 10 grams. One salad helping would put you over this limit, as would most pieces of fruit. As long as one maintains a reasonable amount of vegetable, salad, and fruit in the diet, combined with the appropriate amount of protein, then ketosis cannot occur and neither can kidney damage.

If you have pre-existing kidney damage or have only one kidney, then it is very important that you consume extra salads and vegetables and keep to the low end of the scale for protein intake.

Is this a "high protein" diet?

No, this is not a "high protein" diet. The average amount of protein recommended for a person (assuming they have no diseases, pathologies, or pre-existing conditions) is 1 gram of protein per kilogram of body weight per day. An average 150-pound (69-kilogram) person should be consuming a minimum of 69 grams of protein a day. This is for the sedentary individual who does no exercise. Thus 20 grams per meal still leaves approximately 10 grams extra for snacks.

If you exercise regularly, then you need to increase this amount of protein per day to help repair muscle tissue and provide energy and hormonal support.

A high protein diet is generally considered 40 to 45 grams of protein per meal, or 2 grams of protein per kilogram of body weight per day. This again is assuming that one is a sedentary individual. So as long as the guidelines are followed, you will not be on a high protein diet – you will only be fueling your body with its requirements for daily life.

5. Is this a "low carbohydrate" diet?

No, this is not a "low carbohydrate" diet. This is an unlimited carbohydrate diet, but a specific type of carbohydrate diet. Carbohydrates include grains, starches, sugars, vegetables, salads, and fruit. Then there are many hidden carbohydrates, such as those contained in sauces and condiments. On this diet you may consume an unlimited amount of vegetables and salads with any condiment you like. You may also consume two pieces of fruit a day.

The limitation of carbohydrates in this diet only applies to grains, starches, and sugars. During stage one, for the first eight weeks, there are no grains, starches, or sugars allowed. After this time period, or when you personally chose to move onto stage two, grains, starches, and sugars are reintroduced. Vegetables and salads remain unlimited in stage two as in stage one, but an increase in fruit and condiments is allowed.

For these reasons, the Naturopathic Diet is not a low carbohydrate diet during the weight loss period (Stage 1) or during maintenance (Stage 2).

6. Do I need to take supplements while on this diet?

The use of vitamin, mineral, and herbal supplementation is a very individual topic. Some people when on the diet consume a wide variety of vegetables, fruits, and protein sources, while others tend to confine themselves to a few favorites. Those, whose diet is more diverse, generally consume a healthier combination of vitamins and minerals than those who continually eat the same foods.

The freshness of the foods one chooses also makes a difference. As the nutrient content of food decreases with oxidation and time (after it is picked), those people who consume more frozen foods or food that has remained on shelves for a while will have a lower nutrient content than those who consume more fresh foods.

There are innumerable other factors that influence the need for and type of supplementation. Amount and type of exercise, pre-existing health conditions, smoking, coffee intake, age, and sex all affect vitamin and mineral requirements.

Because of our increased stress levels and the time constraints placed upon most of us today, it is difficult to always consume foods sufficient for all needs. For this reason, I would recommend a multi-vitamin/mineral supplement for everyone. Individual vitamins and minerals should be taken on an individual basis and should be discussed with your health care practitioner. For more information on vitamin, mineral, and herbal additions to the diet, refer to the chapter on Nutritional Supplementation.

A word of caution: Weight loss supplements should only be used when an individual hits a plateau or has a slower than normal rate of weight loss. They should not be used routinely as a means of losing weight. The use of weight loss supplements should always be discussed with your health care practitioner.

7. Can children follow this dietary program?

Yes, children can follow the Naturopathic Diet. Because this diet is not a low carbohydrate diet, nor is it a high protein diet, it will not be harmful in any way to children. In fact, this is a great dietary program for children to follow. Children require a slightly larger intake of protein to maintain proper growth and development. It is the most important nutrient for a child to get, and the one that is most neglected as they tend to favor pasta and breads. Childhood obesity and non-insulin-dependant diabetes in children is reaching epidemic proportions. This diet will not only help treat, but will prevent these diseases. It will also help to instill healthier dietary patterns for adulthood.

By using the guideline of 1.2 grams of protein per kilogram of body weight, it is easy to calculate the basic protein requirements for your child. For a child who does not need to lose weight and has no symptoms of hyperinsulinemia, only two weeks is required in stage one. Vegetables, salads, and fruit contain a much higher level of nutrients than pasta, bread, and rice. Thus your child will actually be consuming a much healthier diet than before.

Even if the child does need to lose weight, most children do not need to follow the full eight weeks of stage one, as their insulin levels are not usually as high as those in adults. This is due to the fact that they have had fewer years of high carbohydrate consumption. After three weeks on the diet (assuming that your child does not need to lose more weight), try to reintroduce the grains and starches slowly. Keep a watch for the hyperinsulinemic signs listed in the book, such as bloating and fatigue after meals. If these signs appear quickly with only small amounts of carbohydrate, then the child's metabolism has not yet shifted and the child must return to the first part of the diet for another two to three weeks.

The health benefits for the child in adopting the maintenance diet are immense and will follow him or her into adulthood. However, if the child returns to previously high carbohydrate dietary habits, the metabolic changes will be reversed and the health benefits lost.

8. Do I need to stop exercising while on the first part of the diet, or will I be tired during exercise?

No, you do not need to stop exercising during stage one of the Naturopathic Diet. In fact, most people find that their fitness and recovery time improve greatly. The main reason for this is that you are now using your food as fuel instead of storing it as fat so your available energy increases. It is also easier to tap into your fat cells as a fuel source. Muscle is maintained and developed rather than being broken down. During exercise, muscle can be damaged. Protein is the principal component of muscle and is required for repair. So once again this diet is ideal for those who are exercising.

For the first few days on the diet, when your body is not experiencing the sugar highs anymore, you may feel slightly tired. Although those sugar highs are not good for the body and they always lead to a crash afterwards, your body gets used to them. This lack of a sugar high can leave some people feeling sluggish during exercise. Once your body is used to the lower, stable, and normal blood sugar levels, you will find that not only does the energy return, but it reaches higher levels than you had before.

If you are training for an endurance event such as a half or full marathon, changes to the diet must be made. These changes may include shortening the first part of the diet, or allowing grains and starches once a day on those days where training is over 1.5 hours.

Again, changes such as these should be discussed with your health care practitioner. Most endurance and high performance athletes find that their performance is greatly enhanced by following the Naturopathic Diet, whether it is introduced well before the race so the body is in maintenance mode during the intense training and racing, or if they adopt it after the main races are over to prepare for the next season.

9. Will I experience headaches for the first week of this diet?

Headaches are usually associated with dehydration, detoxification, or hypoglycemia (low blood sugar). Protein is a natural diuretic, so it is important to drink extra fluids, particularly water. This holds true for both stages of the diet.

Assuming that you keep yourself well hydrated and consume the appropriate amounts of vegetables, salads, and fruit to avoid hypoglycemia, if you are still experiencing headaches, it is most likely be due to detoxification. As you begin the Naturopathic Diet, you immediately avoid many of the toxic foods like sugars, sweeteners, white flours, processed food, and alcohol. When you decrease this toxic load, the liver automatically begins to detoxify the body as it no longer has to deal with ingested toxins. This may cause headaches, fatigue, and even nausea. The more toxic a lifestyle you led before beginning the diet, the more likely you are to experience these symptoms. However, they are only temporary, and all of these symptoms will rapidly resolve as your body cleans. Drink extra water to help the body flush these toxins. If symptoms persist for longer than one week, you should go see your health care practitioner.

10. Will this diet alter my bowel movements?

Whenever you make a significant change to your diet, there is usually a change to your bowel movements. However, this change is different for everyone. Most people find that when their bowel movements change, they always tend to change in one direction. Some people tend towards firmer stools (constipation), while others will experience loose stools. When starting this diet, you will likely move towards your regular pattern of change. It is important to watch your bowels for these changes and make adjustments as necessary. If the bowels get too firm and you are finding it difficult to have a bowel movement, then begin by increasing water and adding in some flax seed oil (approximately 2 or 3 grams at dinner). Flax seed oil is a natural stool softener and bowel anti-inflammatory. If the bowels are too soft, then you can introduce some acidophilus (2 capsules a day on an empty stomach), the good bacteria that always inhabit the gut. This will help to firm up the stools without causing constipation.

It is important to note that this diet usually regulates most people's bowels very quickly. Although there may be an adjustment period for the first few days, the bowels usually return to a regular pattern quite quickly.

11. Is gas normal after meals on this diet?

Digestive gas is usually an indicator that you are not completely breaking down your food. Undigested food passing into the large bowel is fed upon by bacteria that reside there. The bacteria then produce gas as a by-product.

Your liver, stomach, and pancreas normally manufacture the enzymes required to break food down. Once you ingest food, your body secretes enzymes into the stomach and small intestine to help digest the food into absorbable components. The type and amount of enzyme produced is dependant on the type and amount of food ingested. Thus, if you usually intake a high level of carbohydrate, then your body will be accustomed to producing a large amount of amylase and sucrase. These are the enzymes that break down carbohydrates. If you have not been eating protein on a regular basis, then your body will not be used to producing protease, the enzyme that breaks down protein in sufficient quantities.

When you alter your diet, there is often a lag period between new food intake and the body recognizing that it routinely requires a different amount of enzyme production. During this period of time, you may experience slight gas and bloating. If this occurs in excess and you do not wish to wait the time frame for your body to catch up, you may easily supplement with a multispectrum digestive enzyme product. This product would contain all the different enzymes that your body needs and normally produces to break your food down. You would take theses capsules with every meal for approximately one week to 10 days. During this time the added enzymes will take over the degradation of your food until your body has learned that it must produce a different ratio of enzymes for the incoming food. You do not need to worry that by using these enzymes your body will stop its own production of enzymes or not realize that it needs to change its ratio of enzyme production. Your body does not work like that. Your body will continue to recognize the incoming food and slowly make its own enzyme adjustments.

12. What if I have cancer, can I still follow this diet?

There are many schools of thought when it comes to diet and cancer. Those that are clinically founded include the following:

a. Cancer is less likely to grow in an alkaline pH environment.
b. Cancer is less likely to grow when insulin levels are low.
c. Cancer is less likely to grow with organic foods.
d. Cancer is less likely to grow with a higher fiber diet.

a. Protein, fruit, and sugar, in general, are acidic, while grains, starches, vegetables, and salads are alkaline. Protein is less acidic than fruit and sugar and certain protein sources are less acidic than others. For instance, fish or tofu is less acidic than red meat. So to minimize the acidity level, it would be best to consume more fish, egg whites, tofu, and poultry as your protein sources. Similarly, avoiding sugar and large amounts of fruit will greatly decrease acidity levels. To help maintain more of an alkaline environment, it is important to consume a lot of fresh vegetables and salads. Not only do they contain more vitamins and minerals than grains and starches, they will help balance out the pH from the more acidic protein. By following this plan, there is no concern with respect to pH levels, cancer, and the Naturopathic Diet.

b. High levels of insulin have been shown to increase the sensitivity of estrogen and testosterone receptors in the body. When a hormone receptor is more sensitive, it is more likely that it will bind a hormone. Breast and prostate cancer both show increased growth with increased hormone binding. Recent research has shown that hyperinsulinemia increases this response and therefore increases the risk and recurrence rate of certain cancers. By following the Naturopathic Diet, you will only decrease your cancer risk.

c. Inorganic animal products such as dairy, meat, and poultry are injected with growth hormone to force the animal to produce more milk more quickly or to increase the tissue mass of the animal. It is now well recognized that the growth hormone in these products will mimic the growth hormone in our bodies. When growth hormone level is above normal, it can stimulate the growth of all cells, particularly those that are rapidly turning over. Those cells that are turning over most rapidly are cancer cells (for more information see chapter on organic food sources). It is therefore recommended that you consume only organic animal products. Once again this will eliminate any concern with respect to the growth or initiation of cancer and this diet.

d. Fiber has been shown to bind toxins from the bowel and keep our bowel movements regular. Many people think that grains are the only source of fiber. However, most vegetables and salads are higher in fiber than most grain products. As you are not consuming grains and starches during the first stage of the diet, you default to more vegetables and salads to fill your plate and stomach. This leaves you with a higher than normal level of fiber in your diet, and the fiber is from a much healthier source. So once again, as long as you maintain vegetables and salads in your diet on a daily basis, there is no concern about fiber, cancer, and the Naturopathic Diet.

13. On this diet, I lose weight quickly, then plateau, then lose again and hit another plateau. Why do I not lose weight consistently each day?

Our body becomes very accustomed to pattern and routine. If you have been gaining weight or staying the same weight for quite some time, despite the ill effects that may have, your body actually is used to that weight and used to that pattern. When you change to the Naturopathic Diet, your body will respond to this change by a loss in weight. However, your body prefers to remain static, so it will attempt to acclimatize to the new diet and stabilize metabolism and weight. This is the plateau. This period of time usually only lasts a couple of days and then your body gives in and continues to change. Your weight loss will then continue. Second and third plateaus may occur, and this cycle usually continues throughout the entire program. As long as the plateau only lasts a few days, it is of no concern. This is how most people lose weight. Very few people drop weight every day, which is why you should not jump on a weight scale daily. Try to keep it to once a week, so that you will only see that losses.

If your plateau lasts for two weeks or more, you may be a candidate for natural supplementation to help push you through the plateau and speed up the rate of weight loss. Once again, all weight loss supplements, despite the fact that they are not pharmaceutical in nature, should be monitored by your health care practitioner.

14. How will this diet affect my sleep?

Insomnia or even poor sleep is aggravated and often induced by hypoglycemia (low blood sugar levels). Hypoglycemia occurs when our blood sugar levels fall below normal. This is usually brought about by the increased release in insulin following a meal too high in carbohydrates. On the Naturopathic Diet, blood sugar levels remain normal and constant through the stabilization from protein at each meal. Many of my patients report a much deeper, longer, and solid sleep when on this diet. If you are particularly susceptible to hypoglycemic induced insomnia, then try consuming a small protein snack before bed, perhaps a slice of chicken or a couple spoonfuls of cottage cheese. This will help prevent your blood sugars from dropping too low overnight.

15. Why do I urinate more frequently with this diet?

There are two main reasons why you may urinate more frequently during stage one of this diet. First, your insulin will have a profound effect on the kidneys. When in high concentration, insulin directs the kidneys to hold onto salt. When your body holds onto salt, it will also retain water to balance the electrolyte concentration within each cell. This leads to bloating. As your insulin levels fall during stage one of the diet, there is no longer the stimulus to hold onto this salt. Thus your kidneys freely let go of this excess sodium and simultaneously you urinate out the extra water. This is what causes the extra urination at the beginning of the diet. Once your body has reached a stable insulin level, which should occur within one week to 10 days, the rate of urinations or amount each time will decrease. The second reason for slightly more frequent urination is that protein by nature is a diuretic. It will force your body to rid itself of any excess fluid.

For both of these reasons, it is important to replenish your water or fluid levels so that you do not dehydrate yourself. Drinking extra water will not cause bloating as before because the water will not follow the salt into each cell and cause cellular swelling. Instead, your body will hydrate each cell with the appropriate amount of water and then you will simply urinate out the rest.

16. If I choose only those foods that are lowest in carbohydrate, will I lose weight faster?

The simple answer is yes, as long as you still maintain enough carbohydrate content to prevent ketosis and starvation where you will end up forcing your body to hold onto food later. However, you must keep in mind that if you continually eat the same foods over and over again, you will likely not consume sufficient vitamins, minerals, and other important nutrients that come from a varied diet. It is important to eat a well-rounded diet so that your body is replenished with the appropriate vitamins and minerals each day.

You may find that by eating the same foods repeatedly, particularly with no condiments, that you quickly become bored with the diet. It is here that you risk falling off the diet. Remember, this is not a temporary diet change. These are lifestyle changes you are making here. You want to ensure that you enjoy your dietary choices so that mealtime becomes a joy rather than a chore.

17. Why am I allowed peas, carrots, and condiments on this diet when they contain so many carbohydrates?

You are allowed peas, carrots, and condiments during both the weight loss and the maintenance stage of the diet for two reasons. First, there are so many other carbohydrates that have been eliminated during stage one of the diet that I did not feel it was necessary to remove these as well. I have seen great results with weight loss in my patients despite leaving these foods in. When any diet becomes too restricted, there is a risk of non-compliance. If you do not stick to the diet or you are continually falling off, then there is no point in beginning a diet. Dietary changes need to be simple, adaptable, and easy to maintain. By leaving in some of the sweeter vegetables and condiments, there is a much wider variety of foods to choose from. This in turn helps to ensure the permanent lifestyle changes we are looking to achieve.

Second, peas and carrots contain many different vitamins in high concentration. I feel that their nutrient value counteracts their sugar content, particularly as so many other sugars have been eliminated. Because they are higher in sugar, you may not want to choose them at each meal. Similarly, ensure that you always eat protein at the same time to slow down the delivery of sugar from these foods into the blood.

18. What happens if I cheat?

If you cheat during stage one of this diet, it is important to stop and recognize it as a cheat. Most of us live very busy lives, and there will come a time where following the diet may be quite difficult or impossible. If this happens, sit back and take note of how you feel. Do you feel tired, did you bloat, do you feel slightly unwell? Most people find, particularly if they cheat with junk food, that they may feel ill or just not as well as they did before. This is actually a good lesson to learn as it may encourage you not to cheat again the next time.

However, if it has happened, do not castigate yourself. Recognize that you have cheated and just get right back to the dietary habits you were following – the ones that made you feel so great. You may find that you bloat for the day, but once you restart the diet, then you will quickly urinate out that extra water and feel better once again. One cheat will not alter the metabolic changes we are trying to achieve, but several cheats will either slow the process down greatly or halt it completely. It is important to try to be as compliant as possible during those first eight weeks. This way you can teach your body how to handle those cheats later on with no ill effects.

19. What happens if I have an event that I cannot get out of and I know that they will serve foods that I am not supposed to eat?

Life will always present us with situations where it is difficult to follow the Naturopathic Diet. If you know that you will be at a meal where forbidden foods will be served, try your best to minimize their intake. First of all, do not say yes to all alcohol, grains, and starches at the meal and dessert. Try to pick one. This way you can still participate in the meal but not overdo it. Try to eat more protein with this forbidden carbohydrate. Make the physical size of your protein larger than that of the forbidden carbohydrate. This way you will slow the delivery of sugar and minimize the insulin release. You may still consume unlimited vegetables and salads. Just because you have another carbohydrate available does not mean you are not allowed to eat the "good" carbohydrates. Remember, the vegetables and salads are the carbohydrates with the high nutrient content. You may also want to bring a protein bar with you just in case there is no other protein source available. Consume part of the bar to stabilize your blood sugar levels before consuming the forbidden carbohydrate.

Once again, one meal will not damage the metabolic changes you are undergoing. So relax and then get right back on to the diet the next meal.

Once in the maintenance stage, these dietary indiscretions are more easily tolerated, although to reduce the symptomatic effect of a high carbohydrate meal, the guidelines above remain useful.

20. How long can I stay on this diet?

Essentially, one can stay on the Naturopathic Diet forever. As it is not a low carbohydrate diet or a high protein diet, there is no harm in staying on the diet indefinitely. In fact, it is a much healthier diet to follow as you are only consuming calories with a high nutrient content. Your body will stop losing weight when you reach a healthy weight. However, you may want to consume grains, starches, sugars, or more fruit from time to time. Most of my patients never return to the forbidden carbohydrates as frequently as they are allowed too, simply because they feel satisfied and healthy bringing them in only from time to time.

Remember that this diet is not a short-term solution to achieve a certain weight; it is a permanent pattern of eating. The Naturopathic Diet is not only concerned with weight control, but the prevention of disease and the efficient functioning of our bodies.

Recipes & Menus

RECIPES & MENUS

Preparing meals based on the Naturopathic Diet can present a few challenges. Just as the diet requires a change in how we eat for the rest of our lives, so how we prepare the food we eat will change. Here are some hints, menus, and recipes to get started.

Tips To Make It Easier

1. When cooking a protein source at night for dinner, such as a fish fillet or chicken breast, cook an extra one and leave it in the fridge. You can then use this for your lunch the next day or use part of it as a snack when you get home from work to keep you from nibbling on other foods that are eliminated from the diet. Take time on the weekends to cook and freeze food in single portions so that it is easy to pull out for dinner during the week. Chili, curries, and soups are ideal for freezing.

2. Carry a protein snack such as a protein bar or nuts around with you at all times. If you get hungry or cannot find a protein source for your next meal, then you always have one handy.

3. Eat smaller meals more frequently. This way your blood sugar levels will always remain stable and your food will be digested completely without any uncomfortable feelings.

4. Keep your fluids up at all times. Frequently, the sensation of hunger or boredom may actually be thirst. In these cases, it is much better to drink instead of eating unnecessarily.

5. Do not deprive yourself of calories. This is not a starvation diet. If you are truly hungry between meals, then eat. Just make sure you snack on the allowable foods. If you starve yourself, you will end up slowing your metabolism down and craving more carbohydrates.

6. Do not completely eliminate fat from the diet. You need fat to stimulate the release of CCK, the messenger of satisfaction. Without this you will continually search out food to satisfy yourself, even though you are not hungry.

7. If you have a sweet craving, it is probably indicative of low blood sugar levels. Try to eat some protein with a little carbohydrate first, such as part of a protein bar. Not only will this satisfy the sweet sensation, but the protein in the bar will stabilize the blood sugar levels and relieve the craving.

8. If you tend to snack heavily when you get home from work before dinner, have a small snack on the way home first. This

should raise your blood sugar levels and alleviate the need for snacking when you get home.

9. Eat only what you need. Don't have extra vegetables or protein sources if you are not hungry just because they are the allowed foods. Listen to your body. It will tell you when you have had enough or when it needs more food.

Quick Breakfast Ideas

3 Minute Fruit Smoothie

Ingredients

Protein powder, whey or soya based, approximately
1/2 tablespoons (enough to equal 15 to 25 grams)
8 ounces of skim milk
3/4 of a cup of berries, any type
1/2 teaspoon vanilla extract

Directions

Place protein powder, milk, and vanilla extract in blender (hand held blender or mix master). Slice berries into mixture. Blend drink until all berries and powder are completely mixed into milk, approximately 1 minute.

Any fruit may be substituted for the berries, except for a banana.

Tropical Breakfast Platter

Ingredients

3/4 of a cup of low fat cottage or ricotta cheese
cinnamon or vanilla extract to taste
lemon juice, fresh or from a bottle
sliced pear, melon, pineapple, orange and/or apple, 3/4 of a cup in total

Directions

Place cottage or ricotta cheese in bowl. Sprinkle cinnamon or vanilla extract on top of cheese for extra flavor. Place sliced fruit beside cheese for dipping and sprinkle lemon juice if you wish on top of fruit.

Light and Fluffy Eggs

Ingredients

    1 whole egg and 3–4 tablespoons of egg whites

    5 tablespoons of skim or 1% milk

    salt and pepper

    1 teaspoon of butter

    feta cheese (optional)

    1 piece of fruit

Directions

In a bowl mix eggs with milk, salt, and pepper. If using the whole eggs, discard the yolks before mixing. Place butter in a frying pan and melt. Pour egg mixture into frying pan and sprinkle with feta cheese if you wish. Heat until cooked. A piece of fruit may be added on the side if you wish.

Power Breakfast To Go

Ingredients

    1 protein bar with at least 15–25 grams of protein and only half the amount of carbohydrates

    a piece of fruit is optional

Directions

Open bar and eat. Any fruit may be consumed with this but you may not need it as there are carbohydrates in the bar as well.

The Healthy Diner Breakfast

Ingredients

   2 eggs (eating only one yolk)
   3/4 of a cup of sliced fruit
   salt and pepper
   3 pieces of lean bacon (organic preferably) optional

Directions

Boil eggs in water until they float, approximately 4 to 5 minutes. Peel egg shell off of eggs and discard one yolk. Add salt and pepper to taste. Three pieces of bacon may be cooked in a microwave or frying pan. Dab oil and fat off before eating. Any sliced fruit can be used except bananas.

Leisurely Breakfasts

Mexican Omelet

Ingredients

   1 whole egg and 6 tablespoons of egg whites
   1/2 cup of skim or 1% milk
   sliced mushrooms, peppers, onions, tomatoes (any vegetable
      you wish except potatoes, squash, sweet potatoes, and yam)
   1/2 teaspoon of butter
   feta or cheddar cheese
   salt and pepper
   sliced tofu or organic sausage optional, precooked

Directions

Preheat oven on broil. Preheat frying pan with butter it in. In a bowl, mix eggs (discarding egg yolks if using the whole eggs) with milk, salt and pepper. Add egg mixture to frying pan so that it covers the base of the pan. Sprinkle sliced vegetables and tofu or sausage on top. Allow to cook until bottom is completely cooked. Sprinkle cheese on top if you wish and put under the broiler until whole omelet is cooked on top and cheese is melted.

Succulent Soy Smoothie

Ingredients

　　4 to 6 ounces of tofu
　　1 cup of skim or 1% milk
　　sliced fruit of your choice, berries work best
　　1 teaspoon of vanilla extract
　　1 tablespoon of lemon juice
　　water to thin drink if you wish

Directions

In a blender mix tofu, milk, vanilla extract, and lemon juice. Slice fruit or berries into blender and blend until tofu and fruit are thoroughly mixed in. Test how thick the drink is, and if you wish it to be thinner, add water and blend again.

Spicy Apple Melt

Ingredients

   1 apple

   cinnamon

   nutmeg

   3/4 of a cup of ricotta or cottage cheese

   1 teaspoon of lemon juice

Directions

Preheat oven to 350°F. Peel and slice apple into an oven safe bowl. Add lemon juice and cinnamon on top and mix. Spread cottage or ricotta cheese on top of apples. Sprinkle cinnamon and nutmeg on top and place in oven. Cook until apples are soft and cheese caramelizes with cinnamon and nutmeg.

English Seaside Breakfast

Ingredients

   2 or 3 kippers

   1 teaspoon butter

   salt and pepper

   sliced onions and mushrooms

   oregano, basil, or any herb of your choice

   1 tablespoon olive oil

Directions

Melt butter in a frying pan and place kippers in it. Fry kippers until completely cooked. Place kippers aside and add olive oil to the frying pan. Once heated add onions, mushrooms, and spices. Cook until vegetables are soft. Add any herb, salt and pepper to taste.

Better Eggs Benedict

Ingredients

> 1 whole egg
>
> 1 slice of ham (organic preferably), precooked
>
> 1 tablespoon of butter
>
> 1 tablespoon of lemon juice
>
> 1 egg yolk substitute (egg beaters)
>
> cayenne pepper
>
> salt and pepper

Directions

In a poaching pan cook one egg until egg white is firm and yolk is soft. Set aside with precooked ham. Melt butter and keep it on hand. In a blender place one egg yolk substitute, lemon juice, a dash of cayenne pepper, and salt and pepper to taste. Add melted butter to egg yolk mixture and blend again.

On a plate place poached egg on top of sliced ham. Pour hollandaise or egg yolk mixture over the egg and serve while sauce is still hot.

Quick Lunch Ideas

Crispy Chicken/Tofu Caesar

Ingredients
fresh spinach or romaine lettuce
1 grilled chicken breast (preferably organic),
    or 4 to 6 ounces of tofu
finely sliced parmesan cheese
Caesar salad dressing, from a bottle or home made

If making dressing:
2 garlic cloves
1 1/2 tablespoons of lemon juice
1/4 cup of olive oil
1 teaspoon mustard (Dijon preferably)
1/2 teaspoon of chopped anchovy (optional)

Directions
Place washed lettuce in a bowl. Slice grilled chicken or tofu (you can make these the night before) on top of salad. Pour dressing over top and toss throughout salad. Place sliced parmesan cheese on top and serve.

If making dressing, mix all the above dressing ingredients in a blender or with a fork, and mix until it forms a smooth liquid.

The Bunless Burger

Ingredients

   1 chicken, beef (both preferably organic) or soya burger

   romaine lettuce

   1/2 sliced tomato

   1 slice of cheese

   any condiments you wish

Directions

Cook chicken, beef, or tofu burger in a non-stick frying pan, no butter or oil necessary. Again, you can have these cooked from the night before waiting to be used. Place protein burger on a bed of lettuce. On top of burger add sliced tomatoes, cheese and any condiment you wish. This type of burger requires a fork and knife.

Summer Salad

Ingredients for Tuna Salad

   4 to 6 ounces of tuna packed in water

   pepper and salt

   one chopped green onion

   1 tablespoon of low fat mayonnaise

   1 teaspoon of balsamic vinegar

   spinach or romaine lettuce

   salad dressing of your choice

Ingredients for Egg Salad

   2 boiled egg whites and 1 cooked egg yolk

   1 tablespoon of low fat mayonnaise

   salt and pepper

   1 chopped green onion

   spinach or romaine lettuce

Directions

Place tuna or chopped hard boiled eggs in a boil. Add mayonnaise, salt and pepper, and chopped onion. If making the tuna salad add balsamic vinegar as well. Mix all ingredients together and place over top a bed a lettuce. Add any dressing you wish.

Quick Fix Salad

Ingredients

   2 tablespoons or 15 –25 grams worth of protein powder
      (whey or soya preferably)

   1 cup of skim or 1% milk

   or

   1 protein bar with at least 15–25 grams of protein and half the
      amount of carbohydrates

   spinach or romaine lettuce

   sliced carrots, onion, peppers, mushrooms or other vegetables
      that you wish

   feta cheese (optional)

   any dressing you choose

Directions

Blend up protein powder and milk in a mixer until smooth. On the side mix lettuce and vegetables together. Sprinkle dressing and feta cheese over top and toss until dressing covers entire salad.

Hearty, Healthy Soup

Ingredients

 2 cups vegetable or chicken stock
 any sliced vegetables you wish with the exception of potatoes
  or other eliminated vegetable
 1 sliced chicken breast (preferably organic)
  or 4 to 6 ounces of cubed tofu
 1/2 chopped garlic clove
 salt and pepper
 1/2 teaspoon basil or thyme

Directions

Bring vegetable or chicken stock with sliced vegetables to a boil. Lower heat and add spices, salt and pepper and garlic. Simmer for one hour. This can be made ahead of time and placed in freezer or fridge.

Leisurely Lunches

Wild West Chili

Ingredients

1 pound of ground beef (preferably organic) or extra firm tofu.
2 onions
2 red peppers
1 cup mushroom
1 cup of kidney beans
3 cups of crushed tomatoes
2 tablespoons of tomato paste
1 teaspoon of chili powder
1 teaspoon of oregano
3 crushed garlic cloves
1 bay leaf
salt and pepper to taste
2 tablespoons of olive oil
1 cup water

Directions

In a large pot heat olive oil, garlic, chopped onion, and ground beef or tofu. Heat until beef is completely brown or tofu cooked, and onions are soft. Add crushed tomatoes, tomato paste, peppers, kidney beans, mushrooms, and water. Stir until mixed together and add spices. Bring to a boil and then reduce heat. Cover and let simmer for 40 minutes.

Fantastic Fajitas: Chicken, Egg, or Tofu

Ingredients

> 2 large cabbage leaves
> 1 chicken breast or 1 hard boiled egg or 4 ounces of
>   extra firm tofu
> 1/4 cup shredded cheese
> 1/2 chopped tomato
> 1/4 cup hummus
> any other vegetable you wish

Directions

Lay cabbage leaves out flat. Spread hummus over leaves. Place sliced chicken or chopped tofu or egg on top. Sprinkle with shredded cheese, chopped tomato and any other chopped vegetable or spice you like. Fold cabbage leaves over into a wrap.

Crustless Quiche

Ingredients

> 3 egg whites and 1 egg yolk
> 1 tablespoon of butter
> 1/3 cup of shredded cheese
> 2 slices of ham
> 1/2 cup of chopped spinach
> salt and pepper to taste

Directions

Preheat oven to 350°F. Beat eggs, butter, spinach, and salt and pepper together. Chop the ham slices into small pieces and add it to the egg mixture. Pour mixture into a small baking bowl or pan and bake for 30 minutes or until cooked (when a fork can be inserted and pulled out clean with no liquid on it).

Special Spicy Stir Fry

Ingredients

    1 chicken breast or 4 to 6 ounces of extra firm tofu
    1 onion
    1 medium carrots
    1/2 red or green pepper
    1/2 cup mushrooms
    1 1/2 tablespoons of spicy Thai sauce
    2 cups of bean sprouts
    1 tablespoon of olive oil
    any other vegetable of your choice
    1 crushed garlic clove

Directions

In a frying pan heat olive oil and crushed garlic. Cut chicken or tofu into small chunks and fry until completely cooked. Chop all vegetables and add onions and carrots first. Let them soften slightly as they require more time to cook than the other vegetables. Then add mushrooms and peppers and any other allowed vegetable that you like into the pan. Sprinkle Thai sauce on top and stir continuously until all vegetables are soft. Place stir fry on a bed of bean sprouts and serve. You may substitute spicy Thai sauce for any seasoning or sauce you wish. Other suggestions are peanut sauce, honey-mustard glaze, black bean sauce, soya sauce, or any stir fry sauce you prefer.

Seattle Seafood Salad

Ingredients

   1/2 cup of peeled and cooked shrimp

   1/2 cup of flaked crab or salmon

   1/2 cup of steamed snow peas

   1/2 cup of chopped red peppers

   spinach or romaine lettuce

Dressing

   1 tablespoon of low fat mayonnaise

   1 tablespoon of low fat plain yogurt

   1/2 teaspoon of curry powder

   1 teaspoon of lime juice

   1/4 teaspoon of ginger (grated or powder)

   salt and pepper to taste

Directions

To make the dressing, mix mayonnaise, yogurt, lime juice, curry, and ginger in a small cup. Beat with a fork until well mixed. Add salt and pepper to taste.

Toss all the seafood, snow peas, and peppers over lettuce. Pour dressing over top and toss until dressing covers all of the salad.

Quick Dinner Ideas

Tuna Teaser

Ingredients

4 to 6 ounces of tuna packed in water
1 tablespoon of low fat mayonnaise
1 chopped green onion
1 chopped celery stick
salt and pepper to taste
1 thin slice of extra firm tofu
2 slices of low fat mozzarella cheese

Directions

Preheat oven to 350°F. In a bowl mix tuna, mayonnaise, onion, celery, and salt and pepper. Stir until thoroughly mixed. Spoon out tuna mixture on slice of tofu. Place cheese slices on top of tuna and put in oven for 15 minutes. Then place under grill for 1 minute if cheese is not melted.

Outback Bar-B-Que

Ingredients

1 chicken breast (preferably organic)
1 green pepper
1 onion
1 zucchini
1 1/2 tablespoons of olive oil
2 crushed garlic cloves
1 tablespoon of lemon juice

2 tablespoons of balsamic vinegar

salt and pepper to taste

1 tablespoon of bar-b-que sauce

Directions

Slice vegetables into long strip and put in pan. Mix olive oil, balsamic vinegar, garlic, lemon juice, and salt and pepper together in a cup. Pour over vegetables and toss vegetables so that they are completely covered in dressing. Pour bar-b-que sauce over chicken. Place on grill or bar-b-que until chicken is thoroughly cooked and vegetables are soft. Note, chicken should be put on grill at least 10 to 15 minutes before vegetables as it takes longer to cook.

Oriental Tofu Salad

Ingredients

4 to 6 ounces of extra firm tofu

spinach or romaine lettuce

1/2 red onion

1/2 cup of mandarin orange slices

1/3 cup of feta cheese

1/3 cup of sliced almonds

1/4 cup of orange juice

1 1/2 tablespoons of olive oil

1 1/2 tablespoons of white vinegar

1 crushed garlic clove

salt and pepper to taste

Directions

In a cup mix olive oil, balsamic vinegar, orange juice, garlic, and salt and pepper. If tofu is not cooked already, place it in a frying pan with a little olive oil and heat it until cooked. Then cut tofu into small cubes and place on top of salad. Sprinkle the feta cheese, almonds, red onion, and oranges. Pour dressing over top and toss salad until dressing covers entire salad.

Spicy Spanish Scrambled Eggs

Ingredients

3 egg whites and 1 egg yolk
1/2 cup of skim or 1% milk
2 tablespoons of salsa
salt and pepper to taste

Directions

In a bowl beat eggs, milk, salt and pepper. Pour in non-stick frying pan and start to cook. When eggs are almost cooked, add salsa and stir it through until the eggs are light and fluffy. This may be accompanied by fruit or a salad of your choice on the side.

Granny's Clay Bake Dinner

Ingredients

1 chicken breast or turkey breast (preferably organic)
    or 4 to 6 once tofu slice
1/2 cup carrots
1 onion
1 zucchini
1/2 cup mushrooms
1/2 teaspoon thyme
1/2 teaspoon oregano
1 cup of water

Directions

Preheat oven to 350°F. Chop all vegetables and place in clay bake pot. Add water and spices. Place protein source of your choice in the centre of the pot and cover. Place in oven for approximately 30 minutes or until vegetables and poultry are cooked.

Leisurely Dinners

Santorini Island Pepper

Ingredients

  1 green pepper
  1 cup of ground beef (preferably organic) or 2 egg whites
  1 chopped green onion
  1/3 cup mushrooms
  1/3 cup zucchini
  1 medium carrot
  1 crushed garlic clove
  salt and pepper to taste
  2 slices of low fat mozzarella or parmesan cheese

Directions

In a non-stick frying pan place chopped vegetables, except the green pepper, and cook them until they are soft. Add garlic, salt and pepper, and any other spice you wish. In another pan, heat beef or egg whites until completely cooked. Mix the vegetables with the protein source of your choice. Cut the top of the green pepper off and fill the pepper with the cooked vegetable/protein mixture. Place in oven at 350°F and cook for 20 minutes. Just before it is done place the cheese on the top of the pepper and put under the broiler until cheese is melted.

Taj Mahal Chicken or Tofu Dinner

Ingredients

   1 chicken breast (preferably organic)
      or 4 to 6 ounces of extra firm tofu
   1 onion
   1 tablespoon of butter
   1 1/2 tablespoons of flour
   1/2 cup of green peas
   1/4 cup of cashews
   1 tablespoon of curry
   1 teaspoon of cumin
   1 crushed garlic clove
   1 1/2 cups of skim or 1% milk

Directions

Cut tofu or chicken into small cubes. Place protein source of choice with vegetables in a frying pan and heat until cooked thoroughly. In a separate pot, melt butter, add the flour, and make into a paste. Slowly stir in milk over heat until flour paste in dissolved. Add curry, cumin, and garlic and let sit for five minutes. Then pour the curry sauce over the protein and vegetables. Add the cashews and let simmer on low heat for another 5 minutes.

Tofu Ratatouille

Ingredients

1/2 eggplant

1 zucchini

1 medium carrot

1 onion

1/2 cup green pepper

2 tablespoons of olive oil

2 large tomatoes

2 crushed garlic cloves

1 teaspoon of oregano

salt and pepper to taste

4 to 6 ounces of extra firm tofu

Directions

Chop all vegetables except the tomatoes, and place in a non-stick frying pan. Add olive oil and garlic and saute until soft. Crumble in the tofu and add the cubed tomatoes. Stir continuously and add oregano, salt and pepper. Let simmer for 15 minutes. You can add extra water to thin it out if you wish.

Ratatouille can be eaten on its own or poured over bean sprouts. Tofu can also be replaced with 2 egg whites that have been cooked and chopped.

Roast Chicken en Provence

Ingredients

1 chicken (preferably organic)

1/2 cup of sun dried tomatoes

1/2 cup of olives

3 ounces of goat's cheese

1 tablespoon of basil

1 tablespoon of lemon juice

1 1/2 tablespoons of butter

1 onion

Directions

Preheat oven to 375°F. Mix together the goat's cheese, basil, lemon juice, and sun dried tomatoes. Cover chicken with this minute. Place onion inside chicken and place on roasting pan. Pour melted butter over top of chicken. Place chicken in oven and continue to baste as it cooks with the butter that has fallen off it and the natural juices that are extracted as it cooks. Leave to cook for approximately one hour or until the juices run clear when you poke it with a fork.

This may be served with a salad of your choice.

Spicy Thai Salmon

Ingredients

> 1 piece of fresh salmon
> 1/2 cup of lemon
> 1 large chopped tomato
> 1/2 cup of mango
> 1 chopped green onion
> 1 crushed garlic clove
> 1 tablespoon of red wine vinegar
> 1/2 teaspoon of basil
> salt and pepper to taste
> 1 teaspoon of honey
> lettuce

Directions

Place salmon on a plate. Mix honey and lemon together and pour over top of salmon. Allow to marinate for 15 minutes. Place on grill for 8 to 10 minutes. In a separate bowl, mix chopped tomato, mango, garlic, red wine vinegar, basil, and onion together. Add a little water to the mixture if it is too thick. When the salmon is cooked, place salmon on a bed of lettuce and pour salsa mixture over top.

This may be served with a salad or vegetables of your choice.

Children's Meals

Vegetables that any child would love

Cauliflower or Broccoli au gratin

Ingredients

1/2 head of cauliflower or broccoli cut into small bite size pieces
1 tsp of butter
1 tsp of whole wheat flour
1 cup of milk
2 finely chopped green onions
1/3 cup of crumbled cheese (cheddar or chevre)
black pepper to taste

Directions

Preheat oven to 350°F. Bring water in a pot to a boil and add cauliflower. Boil for 2 minutes and then let simmer until cauliflower or broccoli is tender.

Melt butter in a pot and mix in flour until it forms a paste. Gradually add the milk, stirring constantly until mixture is smooth and free of clumps. Add in chopped onion, cheese, and pepper and stir for 2 minutes.

Pour sauce over vegetables and serve.

Crispy Cucumber Salad

Ingredients

1 cucumber

1/2 cup of non-fat yogurt

1 tsp of vinegar (preferably white)

1/2 tsp of lemon juice

1/2 tsp white sugar

1 tbsp of chopped coriander

salt and pepper

fresh mint

Directions

Peel and slice cucumber. Combine yogurt, vinegar, lemon juice, white sugar, and coriander in a bowl. Mix in salt and pepper to taste. Toss sliced cucumbers in with the yogurt dressing and chill for 30 minutes.

Bar-B-Que Broccoli and Peppers

Ingredients

1/2 head of broccoli

1 red pepper

1 yellow pepper

1/2 Spanish onion

1/3 cup passion fruit glaze (may substitute any sauce such as peanut or garlic dressing)

1 tbsp of olive oil

Directions

Cut peppers into long strips. Chop broccoli into small bite size pieces. In a separate bowl place chopped onion, passion fruit glaze, and olive oil. Stir until all ingredients are thoroughly mixed together. Marinade the vegetables in the glaze for approximately 20 minutes. Place on heated barbeque and grill until golden brown or soft.

The Healthy French Fry

Ingredients

   3 large carrots
   2 tbsp olive oil
   1/2 tsp crushed garlic
   pepper and salt

Directions

Peel carrots and slightly steam until a fork can gently pierce the carrot. Cut the softened carrots in very thin slices length-wise. In a separate bowl combine olive oil, garlic, and salt and pepper to taste. On a cookie sheet, place the carrots and drizzle the olive oil mixture over top. Place under a grill until crispy and brown.

Raw Vegetables and Dip

Ingredients

   Choose any vegetable you like – carrots, celery, cauliflower and
      broccoli work well.
   1/2 cup low fat yogurt
   1 tbsp light mayonnaise
   2 tbsp onion or vegetable soup mix (dry)

Directions

Cut vegetables into bite size pieces (the smaller the vegetable, the less chance a child will smoother it in dip, and then re-dip the vegetable. This ensures a good intake of vegetable rather than dip). In a separate bowl, combine yogurt, mayonnaise, and soup mix. Stir until the soup mix is thoroughly mixed in. Let dip sit for 30 to 40 minutes, or until the dried vegetables in the soup mix are softened. Serve in a small bowl with vegetables.

Main Meals Ideas For Children

Sloppy Joes

Ingredients

    1 tbsp olive oil
    1 small onion
    1 green pepper
    1/2 pound lean organic ground beef or tofu
    1/2 tsp of oregano
    1/2 tsp crushed garlic
    1/2 cup of tomato sauce
    1 tbsp brown sugar
    1 tbsp red vinegar
    bread or bun made from high protein, low carbohydrate
        soy flour (optional)

Directions

Chop all vegetables into small fine pieces. In a pan, combine olive oil, garlic, oregano, and vegetables. Cook over heat for approximately 5 minutes. Add ground beef or tofu and stir continuously until beef or tofu is brown and thoroughly cooked. Move contents into a saucepan and add the remaining ingredients. Bring to a boil and then let simmer for 45 minutes.

Slice protein bread and serve mixture over top. This can also simply be placed in a bowl without the protein bread and served like chili.

Children's Chicken Soup

Ingredients

1 chicken (preferably organic)
1 large onion
3 large pieces of celery
4 carrots
1 cup fresh or frozen peas
1 leek
1 tsp crushed garlic
1/8 cup of parsley
1 chicken or vegetable bouillon cube
10 cups water
salt and pepper

Directions

Rinse chicken well and place it in a large cooking tray. You may add onion, clove, or any spice you like at this point. Add a little water and place in the oven at 350°F until cooked.

Once cooked, remove as much chicken from the bone as possible and place the chicken bones in 10 cups of water. Bring to a boil and then let simmer for 20 minutes. Remove the chicken bones from the water. Chop all the vegetables into small pieces.

Add the vegetables, chicken, garlic, and parsley. Once again bring to a boil and then let simmer for 30 minutes. Add salt and pepper to taste. Serve in a bowl.

REFERENCES

Anderson, J.W., Johnstone, B.M., and Cook-Newell, M.E. Meta-analysis of the effects of soy protein intake on serum lipids. *New England Journal of Medicine* , 1995;333:276-282.

Atkins, R. *Dr. Atkins' New Diet Revolution.* New York, NY: Avon, 1992, 1999.

Bensky, D. and Gamble, A. *Chinese Herbal Medicine: Materia Medica.* Seattle, WA: Eastland Press, 1993.

Bethea, M.C., Steward, HL. *Sugar Busters – Cut Sugar to Trim Fat.* New York, NY: Ballantine, 1999.

Boon, H. and Smith, M. *The Botanical Pharmacy: The Pharmacology of Common Herbs.* Kingston, ON: Quarry Health Books, 1999.

Champe, P. and Harvey, R. *Biochemistry.* Philadelphia, PA: JB Lippincott Company, 1987.

Clinical Guidelines as the Identification, Evaluation and Treatment of Overweight and Obesity in Adults: An Evidence Report. National Institute of Health, Obes Res. 1998;6:51-209.

Colgan, M. *Optimum Sports Nutrition.* New York, NY: Advanced Research Press, 1993.

Colgan, M. *The New Nutrition.* Vancouver, BC: Apple Publishing, 1995.

Davis, B.D. Frontiers of biological sciences. *Science,* 1980; 209:88.

Eades, M.R. and Eades, M.D. *Protein Power.* New York, NY: Bantam, 1996.

Eaton, S.B., et al. An evolutionary perspective enhances understanding of human nutritional requirements. *Journal of Nutrition*, 126:1732-40.

Epstein, S. Potential public health hazards of biosynthetic milk hormones. *International Journal of Health Services,* 20(1):1990;3-84.

Epstein, S. Unlabeled milk from cows treated with biosynthetic growth hormones: a case of regulatory abdication. *International Journal of Health Services,* 26(1):1996;173-85.

Erasmus, U. *Fats that Heal, Fats that Harm.* Vancouver, BC: Alive Books, 1993.

Garibotto G., et al. Acute effects of peritoneal dialysis with dialysates containing dextrose or dextrose and amino acids on muscle protein turnover in patients with chronic renal failure. *J.Am.Soc.Nephrol,* 2001, Mar;12(3)557-67.

Goldberg, B. et al. *Alternative Medicine.* Puyallup, WA: 1994.

Greater Boston Physicians for Social Responsibility and the Massachusetts Public Interest Research Group Education Fund. *Generations at Risk: How Environmental Toxins May Affect Reproductive Health in Massachusetts.* Cambridge, MA: Lynn Martin of Martin/VanderLoop Associates, 1998.

Guillette, E., et al. An anthropological approach to the evaluation of preschool children exposed to pesticides in Mexico. *Environmental Health Perspectives,* 106(6):1998; 347-53.

Guyton, A. *The Textbook of Medical Physiology.* 8th ed. Philadelphia, PA: WB Saunders Company, 1991.

Hatfield, F and Gastelu, D. *Dynamic Nutrition for Maximal Performance.* Garden City Park, NY: Avery Publishing Group, 1997.

Heller, R. and Heller, R. *The Carbohydrate Addict's Diet.* New York, NY: Signet, 1993.

Hoffer, A. *Hoffer's Laws of Natural Nutrition.* Kingston, ON: Quarry Health Books, 1995.

Jeppesen, J., Scheaf, P., Jones, C., et al. Effects of low fat, high-carbohydrate diets on risk factors for ischemic heart disease. *Am J Clin Nutr,* 1997;65:1027-1033.

Kendall, P. Syndrome X and insulin resistance. *Nutrition News,* Colorado State University (October), 1997.

Krauss, R.M., Deckelbaum, R.J., Ernst, N., et al. A dietary guideline for healthy American adults: a statement for health professions from the Nutrition Committee, American Heart Association. *Circulation,* 1996;94:1795-1800.

LaRosa, J.C., Fry, A.G., Muesing, R., et al. Effects of high protein, low-carbohydrate dieting on plasma lipoproteins and body weight. *J Am Diet Assoc,* 1980;77:264-270.

LeRoith, D., et al. The role of the insulin-like growth factor-1 receptor in cancer. *Annals New York Academy of Sciences,* 766:1995; 99402-408.

Marks, J. The insulin resistance syndrome. *The Monitor,* 1(3):1996.

Marshall, W. *Clinical Chemistry.* 2nd ed. Philadelphia, PA: Gower Medical Publishing, 1998.

McCroy, M.A., Fuss, P.J., McCallum, J.E., et al. Dietary variety within food groups: Association with energy intake and body fatness in men and women. *Am J Clin Nutr,* 1999;69:440-447.

Merocla, J. *Lower Your Cars and LowerYourIinsulin!* Schaumburg IL: Preventative Environmental Medicine, 1999.

Mesina, MJ, et al. Soy intake and cancer risk, a review of the in vitro and in vivo data. *Nutr Cancer,* 21(2):1994; 113-131.

Messina, M., and Messina, V. *The Simple Soybean and Your Health.* Garden City, NY: Avery Publishing Group, 1994.

Mondoa, E. and Kitei, M. *Sugars that Heal.* New York, NY: Ballantine, 2001.

Montignac, M. *Eat Yourself Slim.* NP: Erica House, 1999.

Murray, Michael. *Encyclopedia of Nutritional Supplements.* Rocklin, CA: Prima Publishing, 1996.

Papa, V., Gliozzi, B., Clark, G.M., MeGuire, W.L., Moore, D., Fujita-

Yamaguchi, Y., Vigneri, R., Goldfine, I.D., Pezzino, V. Insulin-like growth factor-1 receptors are overexpressed and predict a low risk in humans with breast cancer. *Cancer Research*, 53:1993;3736-40.

Robbins, S., Cotran, R., and Kumar, V. *Basis of Disease*. 5th edition. Philadelphia, PA: W.B Saunders Company, 1994.

Robbins, J. *Reclaiming Our Health*. Tiburan, CA: HJK Kramer, 1996.

Rolls, B.J., Bell, E.A., Castellanos, V.H., et al. Energy density but not fat content of foods affected energy intake in lean and obese women. *Am J Clin Nutr*. 1999;69:863-871.

Salmeron, J., Manson, J.E., Stampfer, M.J., et al. Dietary fibre, glycemic load and risk of non-insulin-dependant diabetes I women. *Journal of the American Medical Association*, 1997;277:472-477.

Sears, B. *Enter The Zone*. New York, NY: Harper Collins Publishing, 1995.

Shaw, K. Insulin resistance. *The Lifescience Resource*, 2(3):1997;325-46.

Sites, D. and Terr, A. *Basic and Clinical Immunology*. 7th edition. Norwalk, CT: Lange Medical, 1991.

Warren, P., Porter, J., and Carlson, I.H. Endocrine, immune and behavioral effects of aldicarb (carbamate), atrazine (triazine) and nitrate (fertilizer) mixtures at groundwater concentrations. *Toxicology and Industrial Health*, 15(1 and 2):1999;133-50.

Humfry, C.D. Phytoestrogens and human health: Weighing up the current evidence. *Natural Toxins*, 6(2):1998; 51-59.

Rock, C.L., et al. Nutrient intake from foods and dietary supplements in women at risk for breast cancer recurrence. The Women's Healthy Eating and Living Study Group. *Nutrition and Cancer*. 29(2);24-28.

Volpi, E., et al. The response of muscle protein anabolism to combined hyperaminoacidemia and glucose-induced hyperinsulinemia is impaired in the elderly. *J.Clin Endocrinol. Metab*, 85(12):2000;4481-90.

Welshons, W.V., Nagel, S.C., Thayer, K.A., Judy, B.M., and von Saal, F.S. Health effects of contemporary-use pesticides: The wildlife/human connection. *Toxicology and Industrial Health: An International Journal*, 15(1-2):1999;12-25.